Autoimmune Diseases Explained

A Holistic Approach to Understanding and Managing Autoimmune Disorders

by

Asal Shirazi
B.E.M

The Conrad Press

Autoimmune Diseases Explained
Published by The Conrad Press in the United Kingdom
2024
Tel: +44(0)1227 472 874
www.theconradpress.com
info@theconradpress.com
ISBN 978-1-916966-82-6
Copyright ©Asal Shirazi 2024
All rights reserved.
Typesetting and Cover Design by: Levellers
The Conrad Press logo was designed by Maria Priestley.
Printed and bound in Great Britain by Clays Ltd, Elcograf S.p.A.

Table of Contents

Foreword 9

1. Introduction 15

   1.1 The Immune System and Its Role in Autoimmunity 16

   1.2. Mechanisms of Autoimmunity 19

   1.3 Types of Autoimmune Diseases 22

   1.4 Causes and Risk Factors of Autoimmune Diseases 26

   1.5 Diagnosis of Autoimmune Diseases 28

   1.6 Treatment of Autoimmune Diseases 30

   1.7 Research and Future Directions in Autoimmune Disease Treatment 32

   1.8 Living with Autoimmune Diseases 35

2. Autoimmune Diseases 38

   2.1 Environmental Triggers of Autoimmune Diseases 39

   2.2 Interactions Between Genetic and Environmental Factors 50

   2.3 Prevention and Management of Autoimmune Diseases 51

- 3. Overview of Autoimmune Diseases and Mental Health 56
  - 3.1 Biological Mechanisms Linking Autoimmune Diseases and Mental Health 60
  - 3.2 Psychological Impact of Living with an Autoimmune Disease 65
  - 3.3 Coping Strategies..70
- 4. What is inflammation?...72
  - 4.1 What Are Inflammatory Foods? 77
  - 4.2 Why Inflammatory Foods Matter: Impact on Health 88
  - 4.3 Role of the gut in the immune system 90
- 5. Holistic Management of Autoimmune Diseases Through Diet and Lifestyle 95
  - 5.1 Food Intolerance... 102
  - 5.2 Lifestyle Management 105
  - 5.3 Inflammatory Foods..................................... 108
  - 5.4 Anti-inflammatory Spices include:.......... 109
  - 5.6 What is a leaky gut?..................................... 128
  - 5.7 Deficiencies in dietary vitamins and minerals 137
- Conclusion 140

'Awareness and education is the path to empowerment and control!'

This book is dedicated to my children who have seen me struggle, be moody, foggy, annoying (I have perfected the art), and at times unreasonable due to pain and discomfort yet they have always supported me in my challenges.

It is also dedicated to the Rheumatology and Plastic Surgery teams at the Royal Free Hospital in London, including consultants, nurses, and the admin team, who make sure that I have been looked after selflessly.

I specially want to thank Professor Chris Denton and Professor Ash Mosahebi;

Professor Denton, who has selflessly dedicated his career to looking after scleroderma patients and research and saving their lives. If it weren't for him, I wouldn't be here now.

Professor Ash Mosahebi who has pioneered regenerative medicine and continues to help patients with autoimmune disease and cancer.

PROFESSOR AFSHIN MOSAHEBI

Professor Afshin Mosahebi MBBS FRCS MBA PhD FRCS (PLAST) is a renowned plastic and reconstructive surgeon, particularly recognized for his expertise in complex reconstructive surgeries, cosmetic procedures, and pioneering research in the field of plastic surgery. He holds a prominent position in the UK, serving as a consultant and professor at leading institutions, including the Royal Free Hospital and University College London (UCL).

Prof. Mosahebi has contributed significantly to advancements in reconstructive techniques, particularly for patients recovering from cancer treatments, trauma, or congenital deformities. His research has also explored innovations in surgical technology, including the use of biomaterials, stem cells, and tissue engineering in plastic surgery.

Beyond his clinical work, Professor Mosahebi is actively involved in training the next generation of surgeons and serves as a leader in several professional organizations, including the British Association of Plastic, Reconstructive, and Aesthetic Surgeons (BAPRAS). He is widely published in peer-reviewed journals and frequently lectures at international conferences. His contributions to the field have earned him widespread respect among his peers and patients alike.

About Professor Mosahebi and his fields of work -

Professor Ash Mosahebi is an advocate of research and education. He maintains his position as the deputy editor of the Journal of Plastic, Reconstructive & Aesthetic Surgery and also the author of a number of publications.

Fields of work:
Diseases, Medical Tests and Treatments
- Cosmetic Surgery
- Plastic Surgery
- Breast surgery
- Cosmetic breast surgery
- Dermatological lasers
- Dermatological surgery
- Facial surgery
- Reconstructive surgery
- Rhinology
- Skin cancer
- Soft tissue injuries
- All aspects of cosmetic surgery
- Trauma & oncological breast reconstruction
- Skin cancer & body contouring
- Stem cell technology & tissue regeneration

Foreword

by
Professor A. Mosahebi

In today's world, where medical advancements often dominate headlines, there remains a critical need for awareness about autoimmune diseases—an area of health that affects millions but is frequently overlooked.

This book, *Autoimmune Diseases Explained* offers an in-depth exploration of autoimmune conditions, shedding light on their complex triggers and the profound impact they have on individuals' lives.

It is with great admiration that I highlight the work of Asal Shirazi BEM, whose dedication to raising awareness about autoimmune diseases is both inspiring and essential. Through her commitment, ASAL has become a beacon for many, advocating for greater understanding, compassion, and action in the medical community and beyond. Despite her own daily struggles with eight autoimmune conditions which are debilitating, she maintains a very positive outlook. She uses every opportunity to bring awareness and as a result has made a substantial difference in this area of disease.

Autoimmune diseases, which occur when the body's immune system mistakenly attacks healthy cells, can manifest in various forms—from lupus to multiple sclerosis, rheumatoid arthritis to type 1 diabetes and autism to dementia and Alzheimer's. These conditions often go misdiagnosed or undiagnosed for long periods, leaving sufferers grappling with confusion, frustration, and a sense of isolation.

Often these conditions cause disfigurement, affect mobility and impairment of physiological functions, as well as depression affecting all aspects of the sufferer's life, especially if left undiagnosed or untreated for a long time.

The importance of increasing public and medical awareness about autoimmune diseases cannot be overstated. Asal's efforts remind us of the pressing need for early diagnosis, improved treatments, and, most importantly, empathy for those navigating these invisible battles. Her voice echoes a call for better resources, research, and policies to support those living with these conditions. By fostering understanding, we can help improve the quality of life for millions of people worldwide.

Autoimmune Diseases Explained not only offers insights into the medical intricacies of these diseases but also stands as a tribute to the resilience and strength of individuals like Asal Shirazi, who tirelessly work to ensure that autoimmune conditions are recognized, understood, and treated with the seriousness they deserve.

ABOUT THE AUTHOR

Asal Shirazi BEM is a British humanitarian, entrepreneur, Medical physiologist, scientist, lawyer, and skincare innovator who has made significant strides in the wellness industry. She is the founder of Jeunvie, a multi-award-winning natural skincare brand, and Essentiel Vie, a skincare line focused on mothers and babies. Both brands use botanical ingredients and are designed for sensitive or allergy-prone skin.

Asal established the Autoimmune Support and Awareness Foundation in 2022 after a decade of being a nonprofit and helping the vulnerable.

Diagnosed with Diffuse Systemic Scleroderma in 2005, a rare and life-threatening autoimmune condition affecting the skin and organs, Asal was initially given six months to live. Despite these challenges, she rebuilt her life, channelling her medical and scientific background into developing skincare products that help others with similar skin and health issues. Her work in the field of natural skincare earned her a British Empire Medal (BEM) in 2019, among other prestigious international awards.

In addition to her entrepreneurial success, Asal is a public speaker, mentor, columnist, Aromatherapist, nutritionist, and Skincare Practitioner sharing her health, wellness, and skincare insights through various media outlets.

Despite her own extensive knowledge and experience, she is still coming across so many challenges in convincing the authorities and those who meet her that she suffers from life-limiting conditions that are debilitating. This includes medical staff and authorities set up to give support to sufferers like her.

She decided to use her own experience and knowledge as well as extensive research, to write a book that would help the public in their own management of the conditions. She feels it's important to understand how the immune system works and what triggers it. Using external triggers as a benchmark, we can help ourselves by limiting triggers and hence being more in control of our immune responses.

Allowing empowerment through awareness and knowledge is an important step in the fight against such conditions.

Autoimmune disease awareness is crucial for several reasons:

1. Early Diagnosis and Treatment:

Raising awareness helps people recognize early signs and seek timely medical advice, leading to better outcomes through early treatment.

2. Reducing Misdiagnosis:

Misdiagnosis is common in autoimmune diseases due to their complexity. Awareness educates both the public and healthcare providers and reduces the incidence of Misdiagnosis.

3. Improving Quality of Life:

Understanding triggers of autoimmune disease, symptoms, and possible treatment options can significantly increase the quality of life for people with such diseases. Awareness encourages patients to manage their health proactively with adequate and relevant knowledge.

4. Advancing Research and Treatment: Increased public attention brings more funding towards research, leading to the development of new targeted treatments and potential cures for autoimmune diseases.

5. Reducing Stigma:
Many autoimmune diseases are invisible (invisible disabilities) or misunderstood, leading to stigma or lack of support. Awareness promotes empathy and more support.

6. Encouraging Prevention:
Some autoimmune diseases can be triggered or exacerbated by environmental factors, stress, or diet. Awareness gives empowerment towards informed lifestyle choices, helping to reduce the risk of flare-ups or disease onset.

Increased awareness promotes society to better support individuals with autoimmune diseases and contribute to better health outcomes.

Overall, public education fosters greater understanding, compassion, and action to improve outcomes for those living with autoimmune diseases.

Autoimmune diseases in the UK, as well as globally, are on the rise, leading some experts to describe them as reaching near-epidemic levels. However, they are not typically referred to as an 'epidemic' in the same way as infectious diseases, since they do not spread from person to person. Instead, the increasing prevalence suggests a significant public health concern.

Autoimmune diseases are at high levels in the UK and increasing by 10% annually.

This increasing prevalence of autoimmune diseases is a great source of concern and is reflected in the environmental and lifestyle factors that are ever-changing in society, in particular Western society.

Awareness and diagnostic tools are improving yearly, thus more cases are being identified, contributing to the perception of a rise in cases. However, the impact of the rising number of cases generally, is a challenge for the Public Health sector. These conditions need long-term management and treatment affecting the sufferers and their immediate families.

While autoimmune diseases may not be the single biggest killer in the UK, their rising prevalence and the serious complications they cause—often contributing to other major causes of death like cardiovascular disease and infections—make them a growing public health concern. Addressing this challenge requires greater awareness, early diagnosis, better treatment options, and more research into the causes and management of these diseases.

Asal is hoping that this comprehensive, yet simple explanation of triggers and the workings of the immune system can help bring awareness to allow more self-help and lead to a better outcome for many sufferers, their families and friends.

https://www.autoimmuneinstitute.org/resources/autoimmune-disease-list/

1. Introduction

This comprehensive, simplified guide aims to provide valuable insights and practical advice for individuals navigating the complexities of autoimmune diseases.

Whether you have been recently diagnosed or have been living with an autoimmune condition for years, this book aims to empower and support you on your journey. It is important to explain such conditions' overall cause and effect to help the sufferer control the largely environmental triggers.

Autoimmune diseases encompass a wide range of conditions where the body's immune system mistakenly attacks its tissues, leading to various symptoms and complications. The immune system, which typically protects the body from infections and foreign invaders, loses its ability to distinguish between 'self' and 'non-self'. This results in damage to various organs and systems.

Understanding autoimmune diseases requires exploring the immune system, the mechanisms leading to autoimmunity, the types of autoimmune disorders, their causes, diagnosis, treatment, and ongoing research efforts to uncover new therapeutic approaches.

We will be focusing on the environmental triggers of autoimmune disease, mainly dietary influences which are factors most easily controlled by ourselves.

1.1 The Immune System and Its Role in Autoimmunity

It is essential to first grasp the fundamental workings of the immune system. The immune system is a complex network of cells, tissues, and organs working together to protect the body from harmful invaders, such as bacteria, viruses, and fungi. The immune system is divided into two main components: the innate immune system and the adaptive immune system.

Innate immune system: The innate immune system is the body's first line of defence and consists of physical barriers, such as the skin and mucous membranes, as well as specialized immune cells, such as macrophages and neutrophils. These components are non-specific and respond quickly to pathogens.

Adaptive immune system: The adaptive immune system provides a more targeted response and involves the activation of lymphocytes, such as B cells and T cells. B cells produce antibodies that can neutralize pathogens, while T cells recognize and destroy infected or abnormal cells. The adaptive immune system has a memory component, allowing it to respond more effectively to repeated exposures to the same pathogen.

In healthy individuals, the immune system can distinguish between the body's cells (self) and foreign substances (non-self) through a process called self-tolerance. This process is primarily managed by a set of proteins called major histocompatibility complex (MHC) molecules, which present antigens (pieces of pathogens or cells) to immune cells. When the immune system fails to maintain self-tolerance, it begins to attack the body's own tissues, leading to autoimmune disease

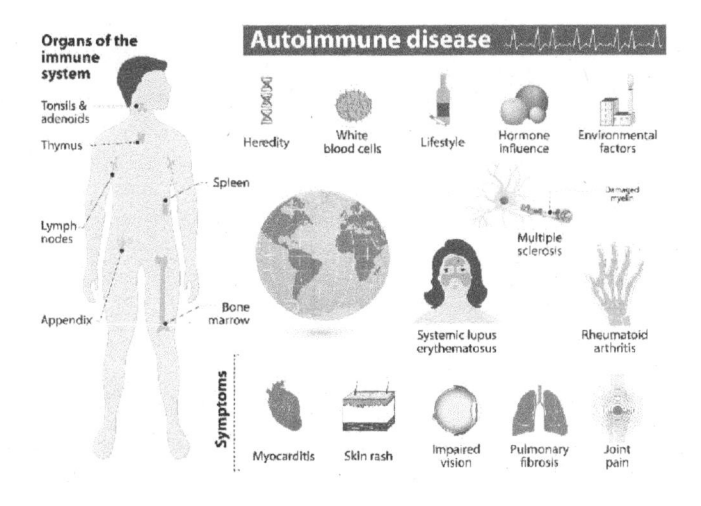

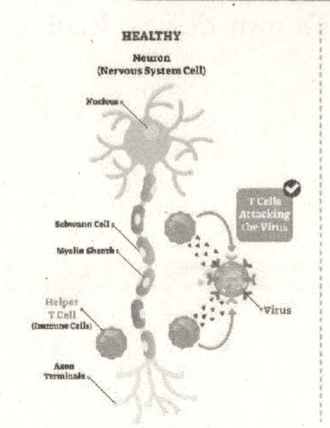

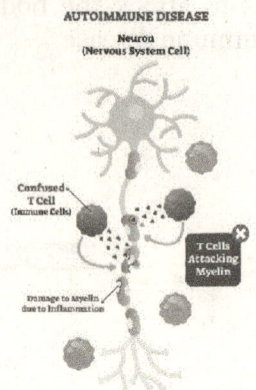

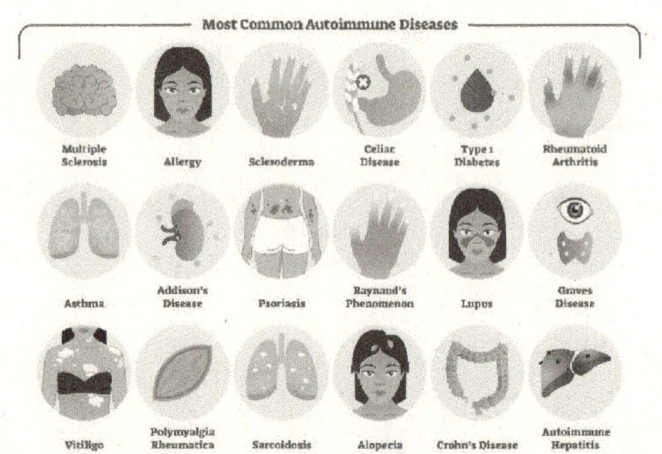

Autoimmune Diseases

HEALTHY
Neuron (Nervous System Cell)
- Nucleus
- Schwann Cell
- Myelin Sheath
- Helper T Cell (Immune Cells)
- Axon Terminals
- T Cells Attacking the Virus
- Virus

AUTOIMMUNE DISEASE
Neuron (Nervous System Cell)
- Confused T Cell (Immune Cells)
- Damage to Myelin due to Inflammation
- T Cells Attacking Myelin

Most Common Autoimmune Diseases

- Multiple Sclerosis
- Allergy
- Scleroderma
- Celiac Disease
- Type 1 Diabetes
- Rheumatoid Arthritis
- Asthma
- Addison's Disease
- Psoriasis
- Raynaud's Phenomenon
- Lupus
- Graves Disease
- Vitiligo
- Polymyalgia Rheumatica
- Sarcoidosis
- Alopecia
- Crohn's Disease
- Autoimmune Hepatitis

1.2. Mechanisms of Autoimmunity

Autoimmunity arises from a combination of genetic, environmental, and immunological factors. The exact mechanism that causes the immune system to turn against the body's tissues is complex and multifactorial. Several mechanisms are thought to contribute to the development of autoimmunity:

Loss of self-tolerance: Central tolerance occurs in the thymus and bone marrow, where developing lymphocytes that recognize self-antigens are eliminated. However, some self-reactive cells may escape this process and enter the peripheral tissues. Peripheral tolerance mechanisms, such as regulatory T cells and checkpoints like CTLA-4, further suppress the activity of self-reactive cells. A breakdown in these tolerance mechanisms can lead to autoimmunity.

Molecular mimicry: In some cases, the immune system may mistake a foreign antigen for a self-antigen due to structural similarities. This can result in an immune response against both the pathogen and the body's tissues. An example of molecular mimicry is seen in rheumatic fever, where the immune system attacks heart tissues after a Streptococcus infection.

Epitope spreading: Initially, the immune system may target a specific antigen, but over time, the immune response can broaden to include additional self-antigens. This process, known as epitope spreading, can exacerbate autoimmune diseases.

Bystander activation: Inflammatory signals during infections or tissue damage can activate self-reactive immune cells that would otherwise remain dormant. This non-specific activation can trigger autoimmune responses.

Genetic predisposition: Certain genetic factors can increase the susceptibility to autoimmune diseases. For example, variations in genes encoding MHC molecules, cytokines, and immune cell receptors have been associated with an increased risk of autoimmunity.

Prevalence

Here's an overview of the statistics and prevalence of autoimmune diseases in the UK:

Overall Prevalence: It is estimated that around 4 million people in the UK (approximately 6-8% of the population) suffer from one or more autoimmune diseases.

Women:

Autoimmune diseases disproportionately affect women, with around 75% of autoimmune disease patients being female. Conditions like lupus and multiple sclerosis are particularly more common in women.

Most Common Autoimmune Diseases in the UK

Type 1 Diabetes
- Prevalence: About 400,000 people live with Type 1 diabetes in the UK, including around 29,000 children.
- Incidence: The incidence of Type 1 diabetes is rising by about 4% per year, especially among children.

Rheumatoid Arthritis (RA)
- Prevalence: RA affects approximately 400,000 people in the UK.
- Age: RA is most common in people between the ages of 40-60, though it can occur at any age.

Multiple Sclerosis (MS)
- Prevalence: There are around 130,000 people living with MS in the UK.
- Geographical Influence: MS is more common in Scotland and northern parts of the UK compared to the south, likely due to environmental and genetic factors.

Lupus (Systemic Lupus Erythematosus, SLE)
- Prevalence: SLE affects around 50,000 people in the UK.
- Demographics: Lupus is more common in women and people of African, Caribbean, and Asian descent.

Coeliac Disease
- Prevalence: Coeliac disease affects approximately 1 in 100 people in the UK. However, it is estimated that only 30% of those with the condition have been diagnosed, meaning many cases go undiagnosed.

Psoriasis
- Prevalence: Around 1.8 million people (2024) in the UK suffer from psoriasis, which is often classified as an autoimmune disease due to its association with the immune system.

Rising Trends

Autoimmune diseases are on the rise globally and in the UK. Factors such as improved diagnostics, environmental changes, and potential genetic predispositions are contributing to the increased incidence of these diseases.

Economic and Healthcare Impact
Healthcare Costs: Autoimmune diseases impose a significant burden on the UK's National Health Service (NHS) due to long-term treatment requirements, specialist care, and hospitalizations.

Productivity Loss: Many autoimmune diseases lead to reduced quality of life and lost workdays, contributing to indirect costs for the economy.

These statistics highlight the growing burden of autoimmune diseases in the UK. Awareness, early diagnosis, and improved treatments remain crucial in managing these conditions effectively.

1.3 Types of Autoimmune Diseases

Autoimmune diseases can affect virtually any organ system in the body, and they are often classified based on the tissues or organs they target. There are more than 80 recognized autoimmune diseases, and they can broadly be categorized into two groups: organ-specific and systemic autoimmune diseases.

In order fully to understand autoimmune diseases, it is essential to first grasp the fundamental workings of the immune system. The immune system is a complex network of cells, tissues, and organs working together to protect the body from harmful invaders, such as bacteria, viruses, and fungi.

Organ-Specific Autoimmune Diseases

Organ-specific autoimmune diseases are characterized by immune responses directed at specific organs or tissues. These conditions typically result in localized damage and dysfunction. Some of the most well-known organ-specific autoimmune diseases include:

Type 1 Diabetes: In type 1 diabetes, the immune system attacks and destroys the insulin-producing beta cells in the pancreas. Without insulin, blood sugar levels rise, leading to hyperglycaemia. Over time, uncontrolled blood sugar levels can cause damage to various organs, including the eyes, kidneys, and nerves. Diabetes 1 would eventually cause death if no insulin were given to the patient.

Graves' Disease: Graves' disease is an autoimmune disorder that affects the thyroid gland. It results in the overproduction of thyroid hormones (hyperthyroidism), leading to symptoms such as weight loss, rapid heartbeat, anxiety, and tremors. The immune system produces antibodies that stimulate the thyroid, causing excessive hormone production.

Hashimoto's Thyroiditis: In contrast to Graves' disease, Hashimoto's thyroiditis leads to the destruction of the thyroid gland, resulting in decreased thyroid hormone production (hypothyroidism). Symptoms of hypothyroidism include fatigue, weight gain, cold intolerance, and depression.

Autoimmune Hepatitis: Autoimmune hepatitis occurs when the immune system attacks liver cells, leading to inflammation and liver damage. If left untreated, it can progress to cirrhosis or liver failure.

Multiple Sclerosis (MS): MS is an autoimmune disease that affects the central nervous system, specifically the myelin sheath that surrounds and protects nerve fibers. The immune system attacks the myelin, leading to nerve damage and disrupted communication between the brain and the rest of the body. Symptoms of MS can vary widely but often include muscle weakness, coordination problems, and vision disturbances.

Myasthenia Gravis: In myasthenia gravis, the immune system produces antibodies that block or destroy receptors at the neuromuscular junction, preventing nerve signals from reaching muscles. This leads to muscle weakness, particularly in the eyes, face, and throat.

Systemic Autoimmune Diseases

Systemic autoimmune diseases involve immune responses that affect multiple organs or tissues throughout the body. These diseases often cause widespread inflammation and can lead to a range of symptoms. Some of the most common systemic autoimmune diseases include:

Systemic Lupus Erythematosus (SLE): Lupus is a chronic autoimmune disease that can affect many parts of the body, including the skin, joints, kidneys, heart, and brain. It is characterized by the production of autoantibodies, which can form immune complexes that deposit in tissues, causing inflammation and damage. Common symptoms of lupus include fatigue, joint pain, skin rashes, and kidney problems.

Rheumatoid Arthritis (RA): RA is a systemic autoimmune disease that primarily affects the joints. The immune system attacks the synovium, the lining of the joints, leading to inflammation, pain, and joint damage. In severe cases, RA can cause deformities and disability.

Sjögren's Syndrome: Sjögren's syndrome primarily affects the glands that produce moisture, such as the salivary and tear glands. The immune system attacks these glands, leading to dryness of the mouth and eyes. However, Sjögren's syndrome can also affect other organs, including the kidneys, lungs, and nervous system.

Scleroderma: Scleroderma is characterized by the excessive production of collagen, leading to hardening and thickening of the skin and connective tissues. It can also affect internal organs, such as the lungs, heart, and kidneys, causing a range of complications.

Polymyositis and Dermatomyositis: These are inflammatory diseases that primarily affect the muscles (polymyositis) and skin (dermatomyositis). They cause muscle weakness, skin rashes, and in some cases, lung or heart involvement.

Vasculitis: Vasculitis refers to a group of autoimmune diseases that cause inflammation of the blood vessels. This can lead to a reduction in blood flow, resulting in damage to organs and tissues. Examples of vasculitis include giant cell arteritis, Wegener's granulomatosis, and Kawasaki disease.

1.4 Causes and Risk Factors of Autoimmune Diseases

The exact cause of autoimmune diseases remains unclear, but it is believed that a combination of genetic, environmental, hormonal, and immunological factors contributes to their development. Some key factors associated with an increased risk of autoimmune diseases include:

Genetic Factors
There is strong evidence that genetics play a role in the development of autoimmune diseases. Certain genetic variants, particularly those related to the MHC (HLA in humans), are associated with an increased risk of developing autoimmune conditions. For example, individuals with the HLA-DR4 allele are more susceptible to rheumatoid arthritis, while those with HLA-DR3 are at a higher risk for lupus and type 1 diabetes. However, having a genetic predisposition does not guarantee that an individual will develop an autoimmune disease, suggesting that environmental factors also play a significant role.

Environmental Factors
Environmental triggers are thought to play a crucial role in initiating or exacerbating autoimmune diseases in genetically susceptible individuals. Some environmental factors that have been implicated include:

Infections: Viral and bacterial infections are common triggers for autoimmune diseases. In some cases, the immune response to an infection can lead to molecular mimicry, where the immune system mistakenly attacks the body's own tissues. For example, the Epstein-Barr virus has been associated with an increased risk of multiple sclerosis and lupus.

Toxins and Chemicals: Exposure to certain environmental toxins, such as cigarette smoke, heavy metals, and industrial chemicals, has been linked to an increased risk of autoimmune diseases. For example, smoking is a known risk factor for rheumatoid arthritis, while silica exposure is associated with lupus.

Medications: Certain medications can trigger autoimmune reactions in some individuals. For example, drug-induced lupus is a condition where certain medications, such as hydralazine and procainamide, can cause lupus-like symptoms.

Hormonal Factors

Autoimmune diseases are more common in women than men, suggesting that hormones, particularly oestrogen, may play a role in their development. Many autoimmune diseases, such as lupus and rheumatoid arthritis, tend to flare up during periods of hormonal changes, such as pregnancy, menstruation, and menopause. Oestrogen is thought to modulate immune responses, and its effects on immune cells may contribute to the higher prevalence of autoimmune diseases in women.

Age

Autoimmune diseases can develop at any age, but they are more commonly diagnosed in young adults and middle-aged individuals. Some autoimmune diseases, such as type 1 diabetes, are more likely to occur in childhood or adolescence, while others, such as rheumatoid arthritis, typically develop later in life.

1.5 Diagnosis of Autoimmune Diseases

Diagnosing autoimmune diseases can be challenging due to the wide range of symptoms and the overlap between different conditions. Autoimmune diseases often present with non-specific symptoms, such as fatigue, joint pain, and fever, making it difficult to pinpoint the exact cause. A combination of clinical evaluation, laboratory tests, and imaging studies is typically used to diagnose autoimmune diseases.

Clinical Evaluation
The first step in diagnosing an autoimmune disease is a thorough clinical evaluation. The doctor will take a detailed medical history, including any family history of autoimmune diseases, and perform a physical examination to assess for signs of inflammation or organ involvement. The presence of characteristic symptoms, such as a butterfly-shaped rash in lupus or joint swelling in rheumatoid arthritis, can provide clues to the diagnosis.

Laboratory Tests

Laboratory tests are essential for diagnosing autoimmune diseases and assessing the extent of tissue damage. Some common laboratory tests used in the diagnosis of autoimmune diseases include:

Autoantibody Tests: Autoantibodies are antibodies that target the body's own tissues. The presence of specific autoantibodies can help diagnose certain autoimmune diseases. For example, antinuclear antibodies (ANA) are commonly found in lupus, while rheumatoid factor (RF) and anti-cyclic citrullinated peptide (anti-CCP) antibodies are associated with rheumatoid arthritis.

Erythrocyte Sedimentation Rate (ESR) and C-Reactive Protein (CRP): These tests measure levels of inflammation in the body. Elevated ESR and CRP levels are common in many autoimmune diseases, indicating ongoing inflammation.

Organ-Specific Tests: In addition to general tests for inflammation and autoantibodies, specific tests may be ordered to assess organ function. For example, blood glucose levels are measured in suspected cases of type 1 diabetes, while thyroid hormone levels are tested in cases of suspected Graves' disease or Hashimoto's thyroiditis.

Imaging Studies

Imaging studies, such as X-rays, ultrasound, MRI, or CT scans, may be used to assess the extent of organ damage or inflammation. For example, X-rays or MRI can be used to evaluate joint damage in rheumatoid arthritis, while ultrasound can assess thyroid size and function in thyroid-related autoimmune diseases.

1.6 Treatment of Autoimmune Diseases

The treatment of autoimmune diseases aims to reduce inflammation, manage symptoms, prevent further tissue damage, and maintain overall health. While there is no cure for autoimmune diseases, various treatment options are available to control the disease and improve the quality of life for patients. The choice of treatment depends on the specific autoimmune disease, its severity, and the organs affected.

Medications
Several classes of medications are commonly used to treat autoimmune diseases:

Nonsteroidal Anti-Inflammatory Drugs (NSAIDs): NSAIDs, such as ibuprofen and naproxen, are used to reduce pain and inflammation. They are often prescribed for conditions like rheumatoid arthritis and lupus to alleviate joint pain and stiffness.

Corticosteroids: Corticosteroids, such as prednisone, are potent anti-inflammatory medications that suppress the immune system. They are commonly used to manage flare-ups in autoimmune diseases, such as lupus and multiple sclerosis. However, long-term use of corticosteroids can lead to side effects, including weight gain, osteoporosis, and an increased risk of infections.

Disease-Modifying Antirheumatic Drugs (DMARDs): DMARDs are used to slow the progression of autoimmune diseases and prevent joint and organ damage. Common DMARDs include methotrexate, azathioprine, and hydroxychloroquine. These drugs are frequently used in rheumatoid arthritis and lupus.

Biologic Therapies: Biologics are a newer class of drugs that target specific components of the immune system, such as cytokines or immune cells, to reduce inflammation and prevent tissue damage. Biologics, such as tumour necrosis factor (TNF) inhibitors (e.g., infliximab and etanercept), are used in autoimmune diseases like rheumatoid arthritis, psoriasis, and Crohn's disease.

Immunosuppressants: Immunosuppressive drugs, such as cyclosporine and mycophenolate, are used to suppress the immune system in cases of severe autoimmune diseases or when other treatments have not been effective. These drugs are often used in conditions like lupus, vasculitis, and autoimmune hepatitis.

Lifestyle Changes and Supportive Therapies

In addition to medications, lifestyle changes, and supportive therapies can play an essential role in managing autoimmune diseases. Some of these include:

Diet: A well-balanced diet rich in anti-inflammatory foods, such as fruits, vegetables, and omega-3 fatty acids, may help reduce inflammation in autoimmune diseases. Some individuals may also benefit from eliminating specific food triggers, such as gluten or dairy, especially in conditions like celiac disease or autoimmune gastritis.

Exercise: Regular physical activity can help maintain joint flexibility, reduce fatigue, and improve overall well-being. Low-impact exercises, such as swimming, yoga, and walking, are often recommended for individuals with autoimmune diseases.

Stress Management: Stress has been shown to exacerbate autoimmune symptoms in some individuals. Techniques like meditation, deep breathing exercises, and mindfulness can help manage stress and improve the quality of life for individuals with autoimmune diseases.

Physical and Occupational Therapy: Physical therapy can help improve muscle strength, flexibility, and mobility in individuals with conditions like rheumatoid arthritis or multiple sclerosis. Occupational therapy can assist individuals in adapting to daily tasks and maintaining independence despite physical limitations.

1.7 Research and Future Directions in Autoimmune Disease Treatment

Ongoing research is critical for improving the understanding, diagnosis, and treatment of autoimmune diseases. Some of the key areas of research and future directions include:

Understanding the Role of Genetics
Advances in genetics, including genome-wide association studies (GWAS), have identified several genetic variants associated with an increased risk of

autoimmune diseases. Researchers are working to further understand the functional role of these genetic variants and how they contribute to autoimmunity. Understanding the genetic basis of autoimmune diseases may lead to personalized treatment approaches based on an individual's genetic profile.

Immunotherapy

Immunotherapy, which involves modulating the immune system to treat diseases, is a promising area of research in autoimmune diseases. While biological therapies have already revolutionized the treatment of conditions like rheumatoid arthritis, newer therapies are being developed to target specific immune pathways with fewer side effects. For example, immune checkpoint inhibitors, which are already used in cancer treatment, are being investigated for their potential to modulate autoimmune responses.

Microbiome Research

Emerging research suggests that the gut microbiome (the community of microorganisms in the digestive tract) may play a role in the development of autoimmune diseases. Alterations in the gut microbiome, known as dysbiosis, have been linked to conditions like inflammatory bowel disease (IBD) and multiple sclerosis. Researchers are exploring how restoring a healthy microbiome through probiotics, prebiotics, or faecal microbiota transplantation (FMT) could be used as a treatment for autoimmune diseases.

Stem Cell Therapy

Stem cell therapy holds promise for treating autoimmune diseases by regenerating damaged tissues and resetting the immune system. Hematopoietic stem cell transplantation (HSCT) has shown success in treating conditions like multiple sclerosis and systemic sclerosis. Researchers are continuing to explore the safety and efficacy of stem cell therapies for a broader range of autoimmune diseases.

Vaccine Development

Vaccines have been a game-changer in preventing infectious diseases, and research is underway to develop vaccines that could prevent or modulate autoimmune diseases. For example, a vaccine targeting Epstein-Barr virus (EBV), a known trigger for multiple sclerosis and lupus, is being investigated as a potential way to reduce the risk of these autoimmune diseases.

Personalized Medicine

The field of personalized medicine aims to tailor treatments to an individual's unique genetic, environmental, and lifestyle factors. In autoimmune diseases, this could involve using biomarkers to predict disease progression and response to treatment. Personalized medicine has the potential to optimize treatment outcomes and minimize side effects by selecting the most appropriate therapies for everyone.

1.8 Living with Autoimmune Diseases

Autoimmune diseases are chronic conditions that require ongoing management. For many individuals, the journey of living with an autoimmune disease involves periods of remission (when symptoms are minimal or absent) and flare-ups (when symptoms worsen). While autoimmune diseases can be challenging to live with, many individuals lead fulfilling lives by working closely with their healthcare providers and adopting strategies to manage their condition.

Support Networks
Support networks, including family, friends, and support groups, can provide emotional and practical assistance to individuals with autoimmune diseases. Connecting with others who have similar conditions can offer a sense of community and reduce feelings of isolation.

Mental Health
Autoimmune diseases can take a toll on mental health, leading to feelings of anxiety, depression, or frustration. It is essential to prioritize mental health by seeking counselling or therapy when needed and using stress-reduction techniques, such as mindfulness and relaxation exercises.

Advocacy and Awareness
Raising awareness about autoimmune diseases is crucial for improving public understanding, reducing stigma, and advocating for increased research

funding. Many organizations, such as the American Autoimmune Related Diseases Association (AARDA) and the Lupus Foundation of America, work to support individuals with autoimmune diseases and promote awareness through educational campaigns and advocacy efforts.

Conclusion

Autoimmune diseases represent a diverse and complex group of disorders in which the body's immune system mistakenly attacks its own tissues. While the exact causes of autoimmune diseases are not fully understood, a combination of genetic, environmental, hormonal, and immunological factors likely contributes to their development.

Early diagnosis and appropriate treatment are essential for managing autoimmune diseases and preventing complications. Advances in research, including immunotherapy, microbiome research, and personalized medicine, hold promise for improving the future of autoimmune disease treatment and ultimately leading to better outcomes for individuals affected by these conditions.

In the meantime, individuals living with autoimmune diseases can take proactive steps to manage their condition, such as working closely with healthcare providers, adopting healthy lifestyle habits, and seeking support from family, friends, and support groups.

By staying informed and taking control of their lifestyle and treatment, individuals with autoimmune diseases can improve their quality of life and contribute to ongoing efforts to raise awareness and support research for these challenging conditions.

2. Autoimmune Diseases

Currently, there are more than 100 autoimmune diseases identified although about 80 are listed and new ones are being identified yearly as a result of various other environmental triggers. Specifically, COVID-19 and its variants.

Autoimmune diseases, such as rheumatoid arthritis, lupus, and multiple sclerosis, are characterized by the immune system mistakenly attacking the body's own tissues. Chronic inflammation is a key factor in the development and progression of these diseases, and certain inflammatory foods can exacerbate symptoms and trigger flare-ups.

Before delving into environmental triggers, it is important to understand the role of genetics in autoimmune disease susceptibility. Specific genes related to immune regulation and inflammation play a crucial role in determining the likelihood of developing an autoimmune condition. These genetic factors include:

Human leukocyte antigen (HLA) genes: HLA genes help regulate the immune system by presenting foreign antigens to immune cells. Certain HLA variants (e.g., HLA-DR, HLA-DQ) are strongly associated with autoimmune diseases like type 1 diabetes, rheumatoid arthritis, and multiple sclerosis.

Non-HLA genes: Other genes involved in immune function and inflammation, such as PTPN22, CTLA4, and IL23R, also contribute to autoimmune disease risk.

While genetic predisposition is important, it does not fully explain the onset of autoimmune diseases. Many individuals with a genetic predisposition never develop the disease, while others without a strong genetic background do. This suggests that environmental factors play a crucial role in triggering autoimmunity in genetically susceptible individuals.

2.1 Environmental Triggers of Autoimmune Diseases

Environmental triggers are external factors that influence the immune system and can initiate or exacerbate autoimmune processes in genetically predisposed individuals. These triggers include a variety of factors, ranging from infections to dietary components, toxins, pollutants, and lifestyle factors. Below, we explore these environmental triggers in detail.

Infections
Infections are among the most well-documented environmental triggers of autoimmune diseases. Both bacterial and viral infections can disrupt immune regulation, potentially leading to autoimmune reactions. Several mechanisms have been proposed to explain how infections may trigger autoimmunity. This fact has been researched and is still under scrutiny concerning the effect of the Covid 19 pandemic and emerging virus variants as well as the incidence of LONG COVID.

Molecular Mimicry

Molecular mimicry occurs when the immune system mistakes a component of the pathogen (such as a bacterial or viral protein) for a similar-looking structure on host cells. As the immune system mounts a defence against the pathogen, it may inadvertently attack healthy tissues that share similar molecular features.

Rheumatic fever: Streptococcus bacteria (the cause of strep throat) have proteins that resemble those found in human heart valves. After a strep infection, the immune system may attack the heart valves, leading to rheumatic fever.

Type 1 diabetes: Some studies suggest that certain viral infections, such as enteroviruses (e.g., Coxsackievirus), may mimic proteins in the pancreas, leading to an immune attack on insulin-producing cells.

Bystander Activation

In bystander activation, an infection triggers a general immune response that inadvertently activates auto-reactive T cells (immune cells that target the body's tissues). This can result in autoimmune damage to the body.

Multiple sclerosis (MS): Viral infections like Epstein-Barr virus (EBV) and human herpesvirus 6 (HHV-6) have been linked to the development of MS through bystander activation. The viruses may lead to widespread immune activation, resulting in damage to the central nervous system.

Autoimmune thyroid disease: Certain viral infections, such as EBV, may contribute to autoimmune thyroid diseases like Hashimoto's thyroiditis and Graves' disease through a similar mechanism.

Epitope Spreading
Epitope spreading occurs when an immune response initiated against a specific part of a pathogen or host cell extends to target additional parts of the host's tissues. This can occur during chronic infections or in situations where the immune system has difficulty eliminating the pathogen.

Systemic lupus erythematosus (SLE): Chronic infections may lead to the release of self-antigens, which are then targeted by the immune system. Over time, the immune response can spread to attack other tissues, contributing to the systemic nature of lupus.

Persistent Infections
Some pathogens can persist in the body for long periods, continuously stimulating the immune system. This chronic immune activation can contribute to the development of autoimmune diseases.

Lyme disease: The bacterium Borrelia burgdorferi, which causes Lyme disease, can persist in tissues for months or even years, leading to chronic inflammation and the potential development of autoimmune-like symptoms, including joint pain and neurological issues.

Dietary Factors

Diet plays a significant role in immune function, and certain foods or dietary components can act as environmental triggers for autoimmune diseases. The interaction between diet and the immune system is complex and involves factors such as nutrient availability, gut microbiota composition, and food additives.

Gluten and Celiac Disease

Celiac disease is a well-known example of a diet-triggered autoimmune disease. In genetically predisposed individuals, the ingestion of gluten (a protein found in wheat, barley, and rye) triggers an immune response that damages the lining of the small intestine.

Gluten: In individuals with celiac disease, the immune system mistakenly targets gluten, leading to inflammation and damage to the intestinal villi. This impairs nutrient absorption and causes a range of symptoms, including gastrointestinal distress, fatigue, and malnutrition.

While celiac disease is the most well-known autoimmune condition triggered by gluten, there is ongoing research into non-celiac gluten sensitivity, a condition where individuals experience symptoms like celiac disease but without the characteristic intestinal damage.

Western Diet and Inflammation

The 'Western diet,' characterized by high consumption of processed foods, refined sugars, unhealthy fats, and low fibre intake, has been implicated in the rising rates of autoimmune diseases in industrialized nations. This diet promotes systemic inflammation and can disrupt the balance of the gut microbiota, which plays a key role in immune regulation.

Processed foods: Many processed foods contain food additives, preservatives, and emulsifiers that can disrupt the gut barrier, leading to increased intestinal permeability (commonly referred to as 'leaky gut'). A compromised gut barrier allows toxins, bacteria, and undigested food particles to enter the bloodstream, which can trigger an immune response and contribute to autoimmune disease.

Sugars and refined carbohydrates: Diets high in sugars and refined carbohydrates can promote chronic inflammation, insulin resistance, and obesity, all of which are associated with increased risk of autoimmune diseases such as rheumatoid arthritis and lupus.

Unhealthy fats: Trans fats and excessive omega-6 fatty acids (found in vegetable oils and processed foods) promote inflammation, while omega-3 fatty acids (found in fish, flaxseed, and walnuts) have anti-inflammatory effects. An imbalance in these fatty acids can contribute to chronic inflammation and the development of autoimmune diseases.

Vitamin D Deficiency

Vitamin D is an essential nutrient that plays a critical role in immune regulation. Low levels of vitamin D have been linked to an increased risk of several autoimmune diseases, including multiple sclerosis, type 1 diabetes, and rheumatoid arthritis.

Vitamin D: Vitamin D helps regulate the immune system by promoting tolerance to self-antigens and reducing the production of pro-inflammatory cytokines. A deficiency in vitamin D can lead to dysregulation of the immune system, making it more likely to attack the body's tissues.

In populations with limited sun exposure or dietary intake of vitamin D, the incidence of autoimmune diseases tends to be higher. This observation has led to the hypothesis that vitamin D supplementation may help reduce the risk of developing autoimmune conditions in susceptible individuals.

Gut Microbiota and Autoimmunity

The gut microbiota consists of trillions of bacteria and other microorganisms that live in the digestive tract. These microbes play a critical role in immune system development and regulation. An imbalance in the gut microbiota, known as dysbiosis, has been implicated in the development of autoimmune diseases.

Gut dysbiosis: Diet, antibiotics, infections, and other environmental factors can alter the composition of the gut microbiota, leading to dysbiosis. This disruption can impair the gut barrier, promote inflammation, and trigger autoimmune responses. Research has shown that individuals with autoimmune diseases often have distinct gut microbiota profiles compared to healthy individuals.

Probiotics and prebiotics: Emerging evidence suggests that probiotics (beneficial bacteria) and prebiotics (compounds that support the growth of beneficial bacteria) may help restore gut balance and reduce inflammation, potentially reducing the risk of autoimmune diseases.

Environmental Pollutants

Environmental pollutants, including heavy metals, pesticides, air pollution, and industrial chemicals, have been shown to disrupt immune function and contribute to the development of autoimmune diseases. These pollutants can directly damage tissues, alter immune responses, and promote chronic inflammation.

Heavy Metals

Heavy metals, such as mercury, lead, and cadmium, can accumulate in the body and have toxic effects on multiple organ systems, including the immune system.

Mercury: Exposure to mercury from contaminated fish, dental fillings, or industrial pollution has been linked to autoimmune diseases like multiple sclerosis and systemic lupus erythematosus. Mercury can bind to proteins in the body, altering their structure and making them more likely to be targeted by the immune system.

Lead: Lead exposure, often from old paint, contaminated water, or industrial sources, has been associated with autoimmune diseases such as rheumatoid arthritis. Lead can impair immune function and promote inflammation.

Pesticides and Herbicides
Pesticides and herbicides, commonly used in agriculture, can contaminate food and water supplies, leading to chronic low-level exposure. Some of these chemicals have been shown to interfere with immune function and promote autoimmunity.

Glyphosate: Glyphosate, the active ingredient in the herbicide Roundup, has been implicated in the development of autoimmune diseases such as celiac disease and multiple sclerosis. Some studies suggest that glyphosate may disrupt the gut microbiota and increase intestinal permeability, contributing to autoimmune processes.

Air Pollution
Air pollution, including particulate matter (PM), nitrogen dioxide (NO2), and other airborne toxins, has been linked to increased inflammation and autoimmune disease risk.

Particulate matter (PM): Inhalation of fine particulate matter, often from vehicle exhaust and industrial emissions, can trigger an immune response and promote systemic inflammation. Studies have found an association between exposure to air pollution and increased risk of autoimmune diseases such as rheumatoid arthritis and systemic lupus erythematosus.

Toxins and Chemicals
In addition to environmental pollutants, exposure to various chemicals in everyday life can act as triggers for autoimmune diseases. This includes

chemicals found in household products, personal care items, and occupational settings.

Bisphenol A (BPA)
BPA is a chemical commonly found in plastics, including food containers, water bottles, and the lining of canned foods. It is an endocrine disruptor, meaning it can interfere with hormone function and immune regulation.

BPA and autoimmunity: Studies suggest that BPA exposure may contribute to autoimmune diseases such as lupus and rheumatoid arthritis by promoting inflammation and disrupting immune tolerance.

Phthalates
Phthalates are chemicals used to make plastics flexible and are found in many household and personal care products, including shampoos, lotions, and detergents.

Phthalates and immune disruption: Phthalate exposure has been linked to immune dysregulation, inflammation, and increased risk of autoimmune diseases. These chemicals may interfere with normal immune signalling and promote chronic inflammation.

Stress and Psychological Factors
Chronic stress and psychological factors are increasingly recognized as important environmental triggers of autoimmune diseases. Stress can have profound effects on the immune system, influencing both the onset and progression of autoimmune conditions.

The Role of Stress in Autoimmunity

Chronic stress can lead to dysregulation of the hypothalamic-pituitary-adrenal (HPA) axis, which plays a key role in controlling the body's stress response. This dysregulation can result in increased production of stress hormones like cortisol, which can impair immune function and promote inflammation.

Stress and inflammation: Chronic stress has been shown to increase levels of pro-inflammatory cytokines, which can contribute to the development and exacerbation of autoimmune diseases. Psychological stress has been linked to the onset of diseases such as rheumatoid arthritis, lupus, and multiple sclerosis.

Trauma and Autoimmune Disease

There is evidence that trauma, both physical and emotional, can trigger autoimmune diseases. For example, individuals who experience significant psychological trauma, such as post-traumatic stress disorder (PTSD), may have a higher risk of developing autoimmune conditions.

Stress-related flare-ups: Many autoimmune diseases, such as lupus and rheumatoid arthritis, are known to have flare-ups that coincide with periods of emotional or psychological stress. This suggests that stress management may be an important component of managing autoimmune conditions.

Lifestyle Factors

Several lifestyle factors, including smoking, physical inactivity, and poor sleep, can influence immune function and contribute to the development of autoimmune diseases.

Smoking
Smoking is one of the most well-established environmental risk factors for autoimmune diseases, particularly rheumatoid arthritis and multiple sclerosis.

Cigarette smoke: Smoking introduces a variety of harmful chemicals into the body, many of which can trigger immune responses and promote inflammation. In rheumatoid arthritis, smoking has been shown to modify certain proteins in the lungs, leading to an immune attack on joint tissues.

Physical Inactivity
Regular physical activity is important for maintaining a healthy immune system and reducing inflammation. Conversely, physical inactivity has been linked to increased inflammation and a higher risk of autoimmune diseases.

Exercise and immune regulation: Moderate exercise has been shown to promote the release of anti-inflammatory cytokines and support healthy immune function. In contrast, a sedentary lifestyle can contribute to obesity, insulin resistance, and chronic inflammation, all of which are risk factors for autoimmune diseases.

Sleep Deprivation
Sleep is essential for immune regulation, and chronic sleep deprivation can impair the body's ability to control inflammation.

Sleep and immune function: Poor sleep quality and insufficient sleep have been linked to increased production of pro-inflammatory cytokines, which can contribute to autoimmune disease risk. Sleep disorders, such as insomnia or sleep apnoea, may exacerbate autoimmune conditions by promoting inflammation.

2.2 Interactions Between Genetic and Environmental Factors

While environmental triggers are important in the development of autoimmune diseases, they often interact with genetic factors to determine an individual's risk. In many cases, individuals with a genetic predisposition to autoimmunity may remain healthy unless they are exposed to certain environmental triggers. This gene-environment interaction helps explain why autoimmune diseases tend to cluster in families but do not always manifest in all genetically susceptible individuals.

The Hygiene Hypothesis
The hygiene hypothesis is a theory that suggests the rise in autoimmune diseases in industrialized nations may be partly due to reduced exposure to infectious agents and other immune challenges during early childhood. According to this hypothesis, the immune system requires regular exposure to

certain microbes to develop properly. In the absence of these exposures, the immune system may become overly reactive, increasing the risk of autoimmunity.

Early-life infections: Some research suggests that children who are exposed to a diverse range of microbes early in life may have a lower risk of developing autoimmune diseases. This may be because early microbial exposures help train the immune system to differentiate between harmful pathogens and the body's tissues.

Epigenetics

Epigenetics refers to changes in gene expression that occur without altering the underlying DNA sequence. Environmental factors, such as diet, stress, and toxins, can influence epigenetic changes, which in turn can affect immune function and the development of autoimmune diseases.

Environmental epigenetics: Environmental triggers can lead to epigenetic modifications that either activate or silence specific genes involved in immune regulation. These changes can contribute to the development of autoimmunity in genetically predisposed individuals.

2.3 Prevention and Management of Autoimmune Diseases

Understanding the environmental triggers of autoimmune diseases opens the door to potential strategies for prevention and management. While genetic predisposition cannot be changed, modifying environmental exposures may reduce the risk of developing autoimmune conditions or improve disease outcomes in those already affected.

Reducing Environmental Exposures

Minimizing exposure to environmental triggers, such as pollutants, chemicals, and harmful dietary components, may help reduce the risk of autoimmune diseases.

Air quality: Improving air quality and reducing exposure to environmental pollutants, such as particulate matter and toxins, may lower the risk of developing autoimmune diseases.

Diet: Adopting an anti-inflammatory diet, rich in whole foods, fruits, vegetables, and healthy fats, while minimizing processed foods, refined sugars, and unhealthy fats, may reduce systemic inflammation and support immune function.

Smoking cessation: Quitting smoking is an important step in reducing the risk of autoimmune diseases, particularly rheumatoid arthritis and multiple sclerosis.

Stress Management

Managing stress and improving psychological well-being may help reduce the risk of autoimmune diseases or prevent disease flare-ups.

Mind-body practices: Techniques such as mindfulness, meditation, yoga, and deep breathing exercises can help reduce stress and promote relaxation, potentially improving immune regulation and reducing inflammation.

Immune Support

Supporting the immune system through lifestyle modifications and targeted interventions can help reduce the risk of autoimmune diseases.

Physical activity: Engaging in regular moderate exercise can help regulate the immune system and reduce inflammation.

Vitamin D: Ensuring adequate levels of vitamin D through sun exposure, diet, or supplementation may reduce the risk of autoimmune diseases, particularly in populations with low sun exposure.

Symptoms of HYPOTHYROIDISM

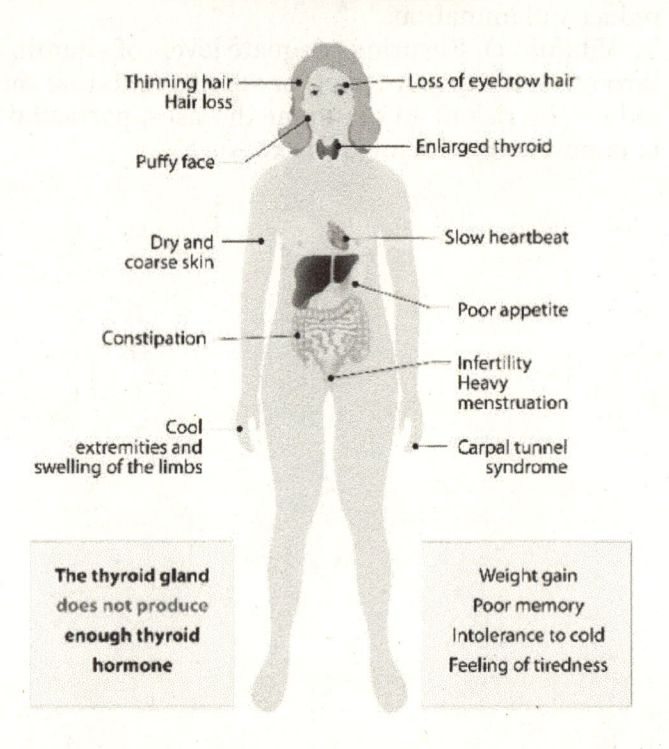

- Thinning hair / Hair loss
- Loss of eyebrow hair
- Puffy face
- Enlarged thyroid
- Dry and coarse skin
- Slow heartbeat
- Poor appetite
- Constipation
- Infertility / Heavy menstruation
- Cool extremities and swelling of the limbs
- Carpal tunnel syndrome

The thyroid gland does not produce **enough thyroid hormone**

Weight gain
Poor memory
Intolerance to cold
Feeling of tiredness

Symptoms of type 1 diabetes

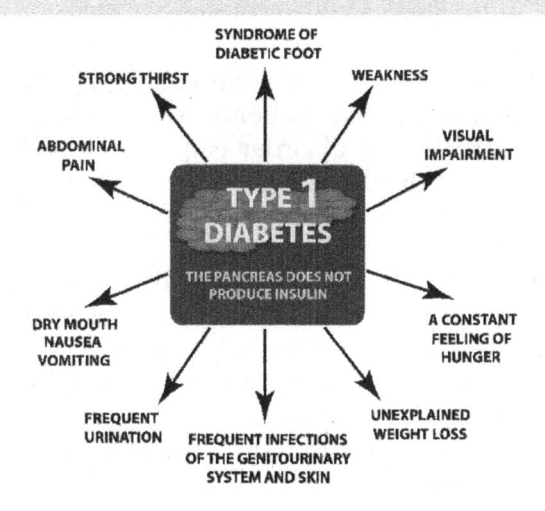

TYPE 1 DIABETES
THE PANCREAS DOES NOT PRODUCE INSULIN

- STRONG THIRST
- SYNDROME OF DIABETIC FOOT
- WEAKNESS
- VISUAL IMPAIRMENT
- ABDOMINAL PAIN
- A CONSTANT FEELING OF HUNGER
- DRY MOUTH, NAUSEA, VOMITING
- FREQUENT URINATION
- FREQUENT INFECTIONS OF THE GENITOURINARY SYSTEM AND SKIN
- UNEXPLAINED WEIGHT LOSS

3. Overview of Autoimmune Diseases and Mental Health

Autoimmune diseases are characterized by chronic inflammation and immune system dysregulation, which can affect multiple organs, including the brain. Mental health issues are common among individuals with autoimmune diseases, and they may manifest in several forms:

Depression: Studies have shown a high prevalence of depression among patients with autoimmune diseases. This mood disorder can be caused by the physical toll of the disease, the stress of living with a chronic condition, and the direct effects of inflammation on the brain.

Anxiety: Anxiety is another common mental health issue in autoimmune patients. It can stem from uncertainty about the disease's progression, fear of disability, and the challenges of managing daily life with chronic pain and fatigue.

Cognitive Dysfunction: Autoimmune diseases can also affect cognitive function, leading to issues such as memory problems, difficulty concentrating, and slowed mental processing. This is particularly evident in conditions like multiple sclerosis and lupus, where cognitive impairment is a frequent symptom.

Fatigue: Fatigue is a debilitating symptom common in many autoimmune diseases and is often linked to both physical and mental exhaustion. It can significantly impact mental health by reducing motivation, increasing irritability, and contributing to feelings of hopelessness.

Sleep Disorders: Sleep disturbances, including insomnia and fragmented sleep, are common in autoimmune diseases. Poor sleep quality can exacerbate mental health problems, leading to increased stress, depression, and cognitive impairment.

Understanding the interaction between autoimmune diseases and mental health requires a holistic approach that considers the biological, psychological, and social dimensions of these complex conditions.

Etiology of autoimmune disease

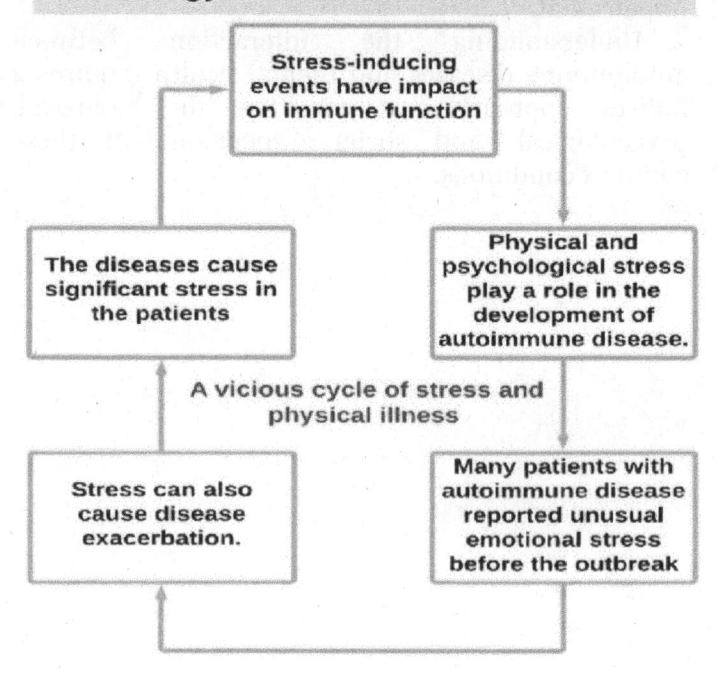

Stress-inducing events have impact on immune function

Physical and psychological stress play a role in the development of autoimmune disease.

Many patients with autoimmune disease reported unusual emotional stress before the outbreak

Stress can also cause disease exacerbation.

The diseases cause significant stress in the patients

A vicious cycle of stress and physical illness

How stress affects the body

BRAIN
Difficulty concentrating, anxiety, depression, irritability, mood, mind fog

CARDIOVASCULAR
higher cholesterol, high blood pressure, increased risk of heart attack and stroke

JOINTS AND MUSCLES
increased inflammation, tension, aches and pains, muscle tightness

IMMUNE SYSTEM
decreased immune function, lowered immune defenses, increased risk of becoming ill, increase in recovery time

SKIN
hair loss, dull/brittle hair, brittle nails, dry skin, acne, delayed tissue repair

GUT
nutrient absorption, diarrhea, constipation, indigestion, bloating, pain and discomfort

REPRODUCTIVE SYSTEM
decreased hormone production, decrease in libido, increase in PMS symptoms

3.1 Biological Mechanisms Linking Autoimmune Diseases and Mental Health

Immune Dysregulation and Mental Health: The immune system's dysfunction in autoimmune diseases can directly affect the central nervous system (CNS). Chronic inflammation, driven by immune responses, can cross the blood-brain barrier and disrupt brain function, contributing to mood disorders like depression and anxiety.

Pro-Inflammatory Cytokines: These immune molecules, such as TNF-α and IL-6, which are elevated during autoimmune activity, have been shown to influence neurotransmitter systems in the brain, including serotonin and dopamine pathways. This can lead to mood disturbances and cognitive impairments, common in autoimmune conditions like multiple sclerosis and lupus.

Autoantibodies and Brain Function: In some autoimmune diseases, the body produces autoantibodies that attack not only peripheral tissues but also the brain. These antibodies may target receptors and proteins involved in mood regulation and cognition, contributing to psychiatric symptoms.

Stress and Exacerbation: Stress is a known trigger for both the onset and worsening of autoimmune diseases, and it also plays a significant role in mental health. The physiological effects of chronic stress can further dysregulate the immune system, creating a cycle where stress exacerbates autoimmune activity, and disease progression worsens mental health.

Immunosuppressive Treatments: While these treatments help manage autoimmune disease symptoms, they can have psychological side effects. For example, corticosteroids are known to induce mood swings, anxiety, and even psychosis in some individuals.

Genetic Susceptibility: Many autoimmune diseases and mental health conditions share genetic risk factors, indicating that individuals with autoimmune disorders may be genetically predisposed to psychiatric symptoms, reinforcing the need for holistic management of both aspects.

This intricate relationship emphasizes the need for healthcare providers to adopt an integrated approach, addressing both the physical and psychological aspects of autoimmune diseases for improved overall well-being.

The link between autoimmune diseases and mental health involves complex biological mechanisms. Immune dysregulation and chronic inflammation can impact the central nervous system and contribute to mental health disturbances.

Additionally, pro-inflammatory cytokines and autoantibodies may affect brain function and neurotransmitter activity, potentially leading to symptoms of depression, anxiety, and cognitive impairment in individuals with autoimmune diseases.

Moreover, shared genetic susceptibility, stress-induced exacerbation of autoimmune activity, and the effects of immunosuppressive treatments on mental health further emphasize the intricate interplay between autoimmune disorders and psychological well-being. These multifaceted biological interactions emphasize the importance of integrated care for individuals affected by both autoimmune diseases and mental health challenges.

I wouldn't go into the medical research evidence for this here as the purpose is to give a generalized overview of the latest findings and to help 'warriors' and their families to have a better understanding of the process.

Inflammation and the Brain

One of the primary biological mechanisms linking autoimmune diseases to mental health issues is chronic inflammation. In autoimmune diseases, the immune system is in a state of constant activation, producing pro-inflammatory cytokines such as tumour necrosis factor-alpha (TNF-α), interleukin-6 (IL-6), and interleukin-1 beta (IL-1β). These inflammatory molecules not only affect the tissues targeted by the immune system but can also cross the blood-brain barrier and impact brain function.

Neuroinflammation: Chronic systemic inflammation can lead to neuroinflammation, where inflammatory cells infiltrate the brain, disrupting normal neural function. Neuroinflammation is linked to the development of mental health disorders such as depression, anxiety, and cognitive decline. For example, elevated levels of IL-6 and TNF-α have been associated with an increased risk of depression in autoimmune disease patients.

HPA Axis Dysregulation: The hypothalamic-pituitary-adrenal (HPA) axis is a critical component of the body's stress response system. Chronic inflammation in autoimmune diseases can dysregulate the HPA axis, leading to abnormal cortisol production. Cortisol, the body's primary stress hormone, plays a significant role in mood regulation. Dysregulated cortisol levels are associated with depression, anxiety, and cognitive dysfunction.

Immune System and Neurotransmitter Changes

The immune system and the brain are interconnected through a network of signalling molecules. In autoimmune diseases, the chronic activation of the immune system can alter the production and availability of neurotransmitters, such as serotonin, dopamine, and glutamate, which play essential roles in mood regulation, cognition, and behaviour.

Serotonin: Serotonin is a neurotransmitter known for its role in mood regulation and is often referred to as the 'feel-good' chemical. Inflammation can reduce serotonin levels by increasing the conversion of tryptophan (a precursor of serotonin) into kynurenine, which is associated with neurotoxicity and depression.

Dopamine: Dopamine is involved in motivation, reward, and cognitive functions. Inflammatory cytokines can reduce dopamine signaling, leading to symptoms of depression, fatigue, and cognitive impairment.

Glutamate: Glutamate is the primary excitatory neurotransmitter in the brain and is involved in learning, memory, and mood. Chronic inflammation can disrupt glutamate signalling, contributing to cognitive dysfunction and mood disorders in autoimmune patients.

Blood-Brain Barrier Disruption

The blood-brain barrier (BBB) is a protective layer that prevents harmful substances from entering the brain. However, in autoimmune diseases, chronic inflammation can compromise the integrity of the BBB, allowing immune cells and inflammatory molecules to infiltrate the brain.

Multiple Sclerosis: MS is a classic example of an autoimmune disease where the immune system attacks the central nervous system, leading to demyelination of nerve fibres. This results in both physical and cognitive symptoms, including depression, anxiety, and memory problems. The disruption of the BBB is a key factor in the neuroinflammation observed in MS.

Lupus: In systemic lupus erythematosus (SLE), a common complication is lupus cerebritis, where the immune system attacks brain tissue. This can lead to a range of neuropsychiatric symptoms, including cognitive dysfunction, depression, and psychosis. The disruption of the BBB allows immune cells and antibodies to enter the brain, contributing to these symptoms.

Autoantibodies and the Brain

In many autoimmune diseases, the immune system produces autoantibodies—antibodies that mistakenly target the body's tissues. In some cases, these autoantibodies can cross the BBB and attack components of the nervous system, leading to neuropsychiatric symptoms.

Lupus and Autoantibodies: In lupus, the presence of autoantibodies such as anti-NMDA receptor antibodies can lead to cognitive dysfunction and mood disorders. These antibodies target brain cells, leading to neuroinflammation and neuronal damage, which manifests as memory problems, depression, and even seizures.

Hashimoto's Encephalopathy: Hashimoto's thyroiditis, an autoimmune disease affecting the thyroid, can sometimes lead to a condition known as Hashimoto's encephalopathy. This rare condition is associated with the production of autoantibodies that attack the brain, leading to confusion, cognitive impairment, and mood disturbances such as depression and anxiety.

3.2 Psychological Impact of Living with an Autoimmune Disease

While the biological factors linking autoimmune diseases to mental health issues are significant, the psychological burden of living with a chronic, unpredictable, and often debilitating condition also plays a critical role in the development of mental health disorders.

Chronic Pain and Mental Health
Chronic pain is a common symptom of many autoimmune diseases, including rheumatoid

arthritis, lupus, and multiple sclerosis. Living with chronic pain can have a profound impact on mental health, contributing to the development of depression, anxiety, and stress-related disorders.

Depression and Pain: Chronic pain is strongly associated with depression. The constant presence of pain can lead to feelings of helplessness, frustration, and hopelessness, all of which contribute to the onset of depression. Moreover, pain can interfere with sleep, physical activity, and social engagement, further exacerbating depressive symptoms.

Anxiety and Pain: Anxiety is also common in individuals with chronic pain. The unpredictability of pain flare-ups, fear of worsening symptoms, and concerns about the impact of pain on daily functioning can all contribute to anxiety disorders.

Pain Catastrophizing: Pain catastrophizing is a psychological process in which individuals experience heightened negative emotions and thoughts about their pain, such as feeling that the pain is unbearable or that it will never improve. This cognitive distortion can increase the risk of developing depression and anxiety in autoimmune disease patients.

Fatigue and Mental Health

Fatigue is one of the most debilitating symptoms of autoimmune diseases, affecting nearly every aspect of a person's life. Unlike normal tiredness, autoimmune-related fatigue is often unrelenting and not relieved by rest, making it a significant factor in mental health deterioration.

Depression and Fatigue: Fatigue and depression are closely linked, as fatigue can reduce motivation, disrupt daily routines, and lead to social withdrawal. The constant battle with exhaustion can leave individuals feeling hopeless, frustrated, and overwhelmed, which contributes to depressive symptoms.

Cognitive Dysfunction and Fatigue: Fatigue can also impair cognitive function, making it difficult to concentrate, remember things, or think clearly. This cognitive 'fog' can increase frustration and anxiety, particularly in individuals who are used to being mentally sharp and productive.

Social Isolation and Fatigue: Fatigue can lead to social isolation, as individuals may not have the energy to engage in social activities or maintain relationships. This isolation can contribute to feelings of loneliness, depression, and anxiety.

Fear and Uncertainty About the Future

Autoimmune diseases are often unpredictable, with periods of remission followed by flare-ups of symptoms. This uncertainty about the future can contribute to chronic stress, anxiety, and depression.

Anxiety and Uncertainty:

Living with an autoimmune condition often brings significant fear and uncertainty about the future, as these diseases are typically chronic, and unpredictable, and can have wide-ranging impacts on health and quality of life. Here are some of the common fears and challenges people face when dealing with an autoimmune disease:

Fear of Disease Progression

Unpredictable Flares: Many autoimmune conditions, such as lupus or rheumatoid arthritis, are characterized by periods of remission followed by sudden flares. This unpredictability makes it hard for individuals to plan for the future, leading to anxiety about when the next flare-up might occur.

Progressive Nature: Some autoimmune diseases, like multiple sclerosis (MS) or Type 1 diabetes, can worsen over time, leading to fears about disability, loss of independence, or worsening symptoms.

Impact on Daily Life

Work and Career Concerns: People often worry about how their condition might affect their ability to maintain a job or pursue a career. Fatigue, pain, and frequent doctor visits can make consistent work challenging, which may lead to concerns about financial stability.

Social Life: The unpredictable nature of autoimmune diseases can lead to social isolation. Missing events, cancelling plans, and the need for rest can create feelings of guilt and fear of losing friendships or relationships.

Health and Treatment Uncertainty

Side Effects of Treatment: Many autoimmune diseases are treated with medications like immunosuppressants or corticosteroids, which can have significant side effects. People often fear long-term health risks, such as infections, weight gain, or osteoporosis, from these treatments.

Evolving Symptoms: The course of autoimmune diseases can vary greatly. Symptoms may shift or worsen, making it difficult to predict how the disease will impact one's body in the long term. This can create anxiety around the possibility of developing complications or other related conditions.

Fear of Permanent Disability

Some autoimmune diseases, such as MS or rheumatoid arthritis, can lead to physical disability over time. There is often fear about becoming dependent on others for mobility, personal care, or daily activities.

The idea of losing autonomy, whether through mobility challenges or cognitive impairments, can lead to intense fear about what the future holds.

Financial Uncertainty

Medical Expenses: Although the NHS covers many treatments in the UK, the costs of managing an autoimmune disease can still be significant. Individuals may need to pay for certain medications, therapies, or adjustments in their home. This can create long-term financial stress, especially if one has to stop working due to the disease.

Income Stability: The potential for periods of unemployment due to illness, or even early retirement, can leave many wondering if they'll have enough financial support in the future.

Strain on Relationships

Family Dynamics: Autoimmune diseases often put a strain on family relationships. Family members may struggle to understand the condition, and the need for caregiving can shift roles within the household, leading to feelings of guilt or resentment.

Fear of Burdening Others: Many individuals with autoimmune diseases fear becoming a burden on loved ones. This fear can lead to feelings of helplessness, guilt, and a sense of losing one's independence.

Mental Health Challenges

Anxiety and Depression: The uncertainty surrounding autoimmune diseases often leads to mental health challenges. Anxiety about the future, feelings of helplessness, and frustration over the physical limitations imposed by the disease can contribute to depression.

Emotional Rollercoaster: Living with a fluctuating condition means constantly adjusting emotionally to the highs and lows, which can be exhausting and overwhelming.

Quality of Life

Fear of Losing Enjoyment in Life: People may fear that the disease will prevent them from enjoying hobbies, travel, or spending time with family in the future. Over time, chronic pain, fatigue, and other symptoms can lead to a sense of losing control over one's life.

3.3 Coping Strategies

Education and Support: Gaining a deep understanding of the condition and treatment options, joining support groups, and connecting with others who have similar experiences can help reduce feelings of isolation and fear.

Mental Health Care: Therapy, mindfulness, and stress-management techniques are critical for coping with the mental and emotional burden of living with an autoimmune disease. Seeking professional mental health support can help manage anxiety and depression.

Building a Strong Healthcare Team: Having a trusted team of doctors, specialists, and caregivers can provide reassurance and create a plan for managing symptoms and flares, reducing some of the uncertainty.

Focusing on What You Can Control: While some aspects of an autoimmune disease may be unpredictable, lifestyle changes, diet, regular exercise, and good sleep can improve overall well-being and give individuals a sense of control over their health.

Living with an autoimmune disease often feels like navigating unknown territory, with many uncertainties about health, relationships, and the future. Support, education, and focus on the present can help manage these fears and build resilience for the journey ahead.

4. What is inflammation?

Inflammation is a natural immune response that helps the body defend itself from infection, injury, and disease.

While acute inflammation is a protective and beneficial process, chronic inflammation can be harmful and is linked to various health conditions, including heart disease, diabetes, autoimmune disorders, and certain cancers. The foods we eat can play a significant role in either promoting or reducing inflammation in the body. Some foods are known to trigger inflammatory responses, which can contribute to the development and progression of chronic diseases.

This comprehensive guide will explore inflammatory foods, their impact on health, the mechanisms behind their pro-inflammatory effects, and the importance of an anti-inflammatory diet. We will also discuss how to make healthier choices and avoid the pitfalls of a pro-inflammatory diet.

Inflammation is a biological response initiated by the immune system to protect the body from harmful stimuli such as pathogens, damaged cells, and irritants. It is part of the body's natural healing process and is crucial for maintaining health. There are two types of inflammation:

Acute Inflammation
Acute inflammation is a short-term response to injury or infection. It is characterized by redness,

heat, swelling, pain, and loss of function in the affected area. For example, when you cut your finger or catch a cold, your immune system responds by sending white blood cells to the site of injury or infection to fight off harmful agents and begin the healing process.

Chronic Inflammation

Chronic inflammation, on the other hand, is a prolonged and low-grade inflammatory response that can persist for months or even years. Unlike acute inflammation, chronic inflammation can occur even when there is no apparent threat to the body. It is often silent and may not present with obvious symptoms, but over time, it can damage healthy tissues and contribute to the development of chronic diseases such as cardiovascular disease, type 2 diabetes, obesity, arthritis, and cancer.

The role of diet in inflammation is increasingly recognized as a significant factor in either promoting or reducing chronic inflammation. Certain foods can exacerbate inflammation in the body, while others can help reduce it.

Mechanism of Inflammation

It is essential to first grasp the fundamental workings of the immune system. The immune system is a complex network of cells, tissues, and organs working together to protect the body from harmful invaders, such as bacteria, viruses, and fungi. The immune system is divided into two main components: the innate immune system and the adaptive immune system.

Innate immune system: The innate immune system is the body's first line of defence and consists of physical barriers, such as the skin and mucous membranes, as well as specialized immune cells, such as macrophages and neutrophils. These components are non-specific and respond quickly to pathogens.

Adaptive immune system: The adaptive immune system provides a more targeted response and involves the activation of lymphocytes, such as B cells and T cells. B cells produce antibodies that can neutralize pathogens, while T cells recognize and destroy infected or abnormal cells. The adaptive immune system has a memory component, allowing it to respond more effectively to repeated exposures to the same pathogen.

In healthy individuals, the immune system can distinguish between the body's cells (self) and foreign substances (non-self) through a process called self-tolerance. This process is primarily managed by a set of proteins called major histocompatibility complex (MHC) molecules, which present antigens (pieces of pathogens or cells) to immune cells. When the immune system fails to maintain self-tolerance, it begins to attack the body's tissues, leading to autoimmune diseases.

Anti-inflammatory food list

FRUITS
- Pomegranate
- Papaya
- Watermelon
- Berries
- Dates
- Grapes

VEGETABLES
- Brussels sprouts
- Cabbage
- Cauliflower, Broccoli
- Beetroot
- Avocado
- Arugula, bok choy
- Eggplant
- Garlic
- Spinach
- Mushrooms
- Onions

NUTS AND SEEDS
- Chia seeds
- Pumpkin seeds
- Walnuts
- Macadamia nuts
- Flax seeds, Hemp seeds

PROTEIN
- Salmon
- Sardines
- Mackerel
- Tofu, tempeh and edamame
- Black beans
- Chickpeas
- Fava beans
- Lentils
- Eggs
- Greek yogurt
- Shellfish
- Beef and pork tenderloin
- Skinless chicken, turkey

OILS
- Almond / Peanut butter
- Coconut oil
- Avocado oil
- Olive oil
- Algal oil

SPICES
- Cayenne pepper
- Coriander
- Turmeric
- Cumin

oilswelove.com

The Gut Microbiota and Immune Diseases

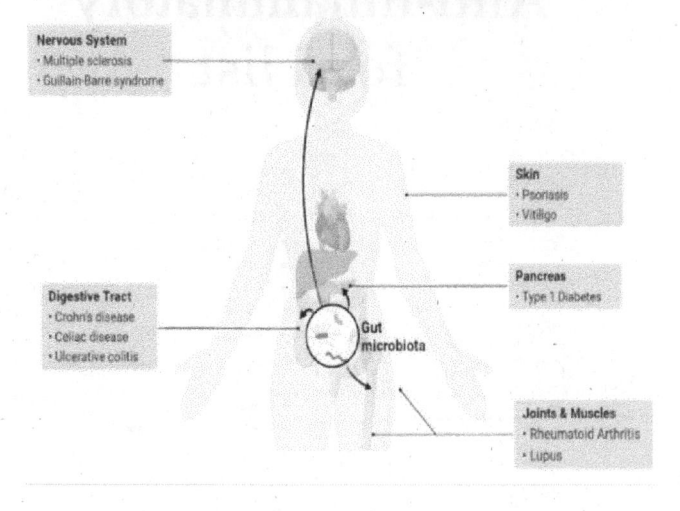

Nervous System
- Multiple sclerosis
- Guillain-Barre syndrome

Skin
- Psoriasis
- Vitiligo

Pancreas
- Type 1 Diabetes

Digestive Tract
- Crohn's disease
- Celiac disease
- Ulcerative colitis

Gut microbiota

Joints & Muscles
- Rheumatoid Arthritis
- Lupus

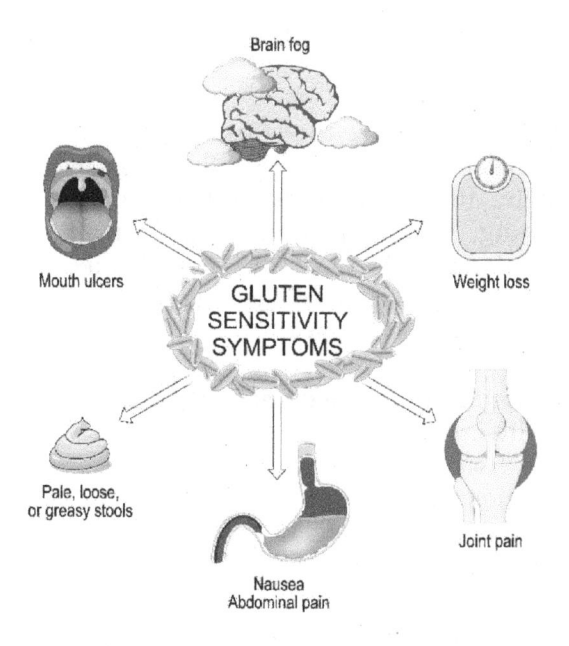

4.1 What Are Inflammatory Foods?

Inflammatory foods are those that can trigger or worsen inflammation in the body. These foods often contain substances that promote the release of inflammatory markers or that cause oxidative stress, both of which contribute to chronic inflammation. Inflammatory foods are typically high in refined sugars, unhealthy fats, and artificial additives, and low in essential nutrients.

Below are some of the main categories of inflammatory foods and how they contribute to inflammation:

Processed and Refined Carbohydrates

Processed and refined carbohydrates are stripped of their fibre, vitamins, and minerals during processing, leaving behind simple sugars that are quickly absorbed by the body. These refined carbs can lead to rapid spikes in blood sugar levels and trigger an inflammatory response.

Examples of Refined Carbohydrates
White bread
White rice
Pastries and cakes
Breakfast cereals
White pasta
Crackers
Sugary snacks and sweets

Mechanism of Inflammation

Refined carbohydrates have a high glycaemic index, which means they cause rapid increases in blood sugar and insulin levels. These spikes can lead to the release of pro-inflammatory cytokines, signalling molecules that promote inflammation. Over time, frequent consumption of high-glycaemic foods can lead to insulin resistance, which is a key factor in the development of chronic inflammation and metabolic disorders such as type 2 diabetes.

In addition, refined carbohydrates contribute to weight gain and obesity, which is closely linked to chronic inflammation. Excess body fat, particularly visceral fat (fat stored around the organs), releases inflammatory molecules called adipokines, further fuelling the inflammatory process.

Sugary Foods and Beverages
Added sugars are found in many processed foods and beverages, and they are one of the most significant contributors to chronic inflammation. Excessive sugar consumption has been linked to a wide range of health problems, including obesity, type 2 diabetes, heart disease, and non-alcoholic fatty liver disease (NAFLD), all of which have inflammatory components.

Examples of Sugary Foods and Drinks
Soda and sugary soft drinks
Energy drinks
Candy and sweets
Pastries, cakes, and cookies
Flavoured yogurts
Ice cream
Sweetened breakfast cereals
Fruit juices with added sugar

Mechanism of Inflammation
High sugar intake can lead to the overproduction of advanced glycation end products (AGEs), compounds formed when sugar molecules attach to proteins or fats in the body. AGEs stimulate the release of inflammatory molecules and oxidative stress, which can damage tissues and cells.

Fructose, a type of sugar commonly found in sugary beverages, has been shown to have particularly harmful effects on inflammation. Excessive fructose consumption can lead to an increase in inflammatory markers such as C-reactive protein (CRP) and interleukin-6 (IL-6). It can also promote the accumulation of fat in the liver, leading to non-alcoholic fatty liver disease (NAFLD), a condition characterized by chronic liver inflammation.

Trans Fats
Trans fats, also known as partially hydrogenated oils, are artificially created fats that are added to processed foods to increase their shelf life and improve texture. These fats are known to be highly inflammatory and are associated with an increased risk of heart disease, stroke, and type 2 diabetes.

Examples of Trans Fat-Containing Foods
Margarine
Shortening
Fried fast foods (e.g., French fries, fried chicken)
Baked goods (e.g., cakes, pies, cookies)
Packaged snacks (e.g., crackers, chips, microwave popcorn)
Frozen pizzas
Processed snack cakes and pastries

Mechanism of Inflammation
Trans fats are known to increase levels of low-density lipoprotein (LDL) cholesterol, often referred to as 'bad' cholesterol, while simultaneously lowering high-density lipoprotein (HDL) cholesterol, or 'good'

cholesterol. This imbalance promotes the development of atherosclerosis (the buildup of fatty plaques in the arteries) and increases the risk of cardiovascular disease.

Moreover, trans fats trigger inflammation by increasing levels of inflammatory markers such as CRP and tumour necrosis factor-alpha (TNF-α). They can also impair the function of the endothelium, the thin layer of cells that lines the blood vessels, leading to endothelial dysfunction, a key factor in the development of heart disease.

Processed Meats

Processed meats, such as bacon, sausage, hot dogs, and deli meats, are often high in saturated fats, sodium, and preservatives like nitrates and nitrites. These foods are associated with an increased risk of chronic diseases, including heart disease, cancer, and type 2 diabetes, all of which involve inflammation.

Examples of Processed Meats
Bacon
Sausage
Hot dogs
Ham
Salami
Pepperoni
Deli meats (e.g., turkey, roast beef, bologna)
Smoked or cured meat

Mechanism of Inflammation
Processed meats contain compounds such as nitrates, nitrites, and advanced glycation end

products (AGEs) that can promote inflammation in the body. These compounds can increase oxidative stress and the production of inflammatory cytokines.

Additionally, processed meats are high in saturated fats, which can raise LDL cholesterol levels and contribute to inflammation in the arteries. Studies have shown that regular consumption of processed meats is linked to higher levels of CRP and other inflammatory markers.

It is essential to first grasp the fundamental workings of the immune system. The immune system is a complex network of cells, tissues, and organs working together to protect the body from harmful invaders, such as bacteria, viruses, and fungi. The immune system is divided into two main components: the innate immune system and the adaptive immune system.

Innate immune system: The innate immune system is the body's first line of defence and consists of physical barriers, such as the skin and mucous membranes, as well as specialized immune cells, such as macrophages and neutrophils. These components are non-specific and respond quickly to pathogens.

Adaptive immune system: The adaptive immune system provides a more targeted response and involves the activation of lymphocytes, such as B cells and T cells. B cells produce antibodies that can neutralize pathogens, while T cells recognize and destroy infected or abnormal cells. The adaptive immune system has a memory component, allowing it to respond more effectively to repeated exposures to the same pathogen.

In healthy individuals, the immune system can distinguish between the body's own cells (self) and foreign substances (non-self) through a process called self-tolerance. This process is primarily managed by a set of proteins called major histocompatibility complex (MHC) molecules, which present antigens (pieces of pathogens or cells) to immune cells. When the immune system fails to maintain self-tolerance, it begins to attack the body's own tissues, leading to autoimmune diseases.

Red Meat (in Excess)
While red meat is a good source of protein, iron, and essential nutrients, excessive consumption of red meat, particularly fatty cuts, has been associated with increased inflammation and a higher risk of chronic diseases, such as heart disease, cancer, and diabetes.

Examples of Red Meat
Beef
Pork
Lamb
Veal

Mechanism of Inflammation
Red meat is high in saturated fats and cholesterol, both of which can contribute to the buildup of plaque in the arteries and increase the risk of cardiovascular disease. The consumption of red meat is also linked to the production of AGEs, which promote inflammation and oxidative stress.

In addition, red meat contains a compound called carnitine, which can be metabolized by gut bacteria into a substance called trimethylamine-N-oxide (TMAO). Elevated levels of TMAO have been shown to increase inflammation and the risk of atherosclerosis.

It is worth noting that not all red meat has the same inflammatory potential. Grass-fed and pasture-raised meats are generally lower in inflammatory compounds and may have a healthier balance of omega-3 to omega-6 fatty acids compared to conventionally raised meats.

Fried and Fast Foods

Fried and fast foods are typically high in unhealthy fats, refined carbohydrates, and sodium, all of which can contribute to chronic inflammation. These foods are often prepared using methods that promote the formation of harmful compounds, such as trans fats and AGEs.

Examples of Fried and Fast Foods
French fries
Fried chicken
Donuts
Fried fish
Onion rings
Fast food burgers
Pizza
Fried snacks (e.g., potato chips, fried cheese sticks)

Mechanism of Inflammation

Fried foods are often cooked at high temperatures, which can lead to the formation of AGEs and other harmful compounds that trigger inflammation in the body. These foods are also high in trans fats, which increase levels of LDL cholesterol and promote inflammation in the arteries.

Moreover, fast foods are typically low in essential nutrients, fibre, and antioxidants, which are important for reducing inflammation and supporting overall health. The consumption of fast food is associated with higher levels of inflammatory markers such as CRP and IL-6.

Excessive Alcohol

Moderate alcohol consumption may have some health benefits, such as improving heart health, but excessive alcohol intake is strongly linked to inflammation and a range of chronic diseases, including liver disease, cardiovascular disease, and certain cancers.

Examples of Alcoholic Beverages
Beer
Wine
Spirits (e.g., vodka, whiskey, rum)

Mechanism of Inflammation

Excessive alcohol consumption can lead to the production of toxic byproducts, such as acetaldehyde, which can damage tissues and trigger inflammation. Chronic alcohol use is also associated with increased gut permeability, allowing harmful substances to enter the bloodstream and provoke an immune response.

Additionally, excessive alcohol intake can impair liver function, leading to alcoholic liver disease, a condition characterized by chronic inflammation and the accumulation of fat in the liver (steatosis). Over time, this can progress to more severe conditions, such as alcoholic hepatitis and cirrhosis, both of which involve significant inflammation.

Artificial Additives and Preservatives

Many processed foods contain artificial additives, preservatives, and flavour enhancers that can contribute to inflammation. These substances are often added to improve the taste, texture, and shelf life of foods, but they can have negative effects on health when consumed in large quantities.

Examples of Additives and Preservatives
Monosodium glutamate (MSG)
Artificial sweeteners (e.g., aspartame, saccharin)
Food dyes
Preservatives (e.g., sodium benzoate, sulphites, nitrates)
Emulsifiers (e.g., polysorbate 80, carrageenan)

Mechanism of Inflammation
Some artificial additives, such as MSG and artificial sweeteners, have been shown to increase levels of inflammatory markers and oxidative stress in the body. Additionally, certain preservatives, such as nitrates and nitrites, can lead to the formation of harmful compounds that promote inflammation.

Emulsifiers, commonly found in processed foods to improve texture and prevent separation, have been shown to disrupt the gut microbiota and increase gut permeability, both of which can contribute to inflammation.

Omega-6 Fatty Acids (in Excess)
Omega-6 fatty acids are a type of polyunsaturated fat that is essential for health, as they play a role in brain function and cell growth. However, when consumed in excess and in disproportionate amounts compared to omega-3 fatty acids, omega-6 fatty acids can promote inflammation.

Examples of Omega-6-Rich Foods
Vegetable oils (e.g., soybean oil, corn oil, sunflower oil)
Processed snack foods (e.g., chips, crackers)
Margarine
Salad dressings
Mayonnaise
Fried foods

Mechanism of Inflammation
Omega-6 fatty acids are metabolized into pro-inflammatory molecules called eicosanoids, which can contribute to chronic inflammation when consumed in excess. While omega-6 fats are necessary for the body, the modern Western diet often contains an imbalance of omega-6 to omega-3 fatty acids, with far more omega-6 fats being consumed. This imbalance can exacerbate inflammation.

To counteract this, it is important to increase the intake of anti-inflammatory omega-3 fatty acids, which are found in foods such as fatty fish, flaxseeds, chia seeds, and walnuts.

4.2 Why Inflammatory Foods Matter: Impact on Health

Consuming a diet high in inflammatory foods can have wide-ranging effects on health, contributing to the development and progression of several chronic diseases. Some of the key health risks associated with inflammatory foods include:

Cardiovascular Disease
Chronic inflammation plays a central role in the development of cardiovascular disease, particularly in the formation of atherosclerosis, where fatty plaques build up in the arteries. Inflammatory foods, such as trans fats, processed meats, and sugary beverages, can contribute to the progression of heart disease by promoting inflammation in the blood vessels.

Type 2 Diabetes
A diet high in refined carbohydrates, sugary foods, and processed foods can lead to insulin resistance, a condition in which the body's cells become less responsive to insulin. This insulin resistance is closely linked to chronic inflammation and is a major risk factor for the development of type 2 diabetes.

Obesity
Obesity is both a cause and a consequence of chronic inflammation. Excess body fat, particularly visceral fat, releases inflammatory molecules called adipokines, which contribute to low-grade systemic inflammation. Inflammatory foods, such as refined carbohydrates and sugary beverages, can promote weight gain and exacerbate this inflammatory response.

Cancer
Chronic inflammation has been linked to the development of certain cancers, including colorectal, breast, and liver cancer. Inflammatory foods can contribute to oxidative stress and DNA damage, which can promote the growth of cancer cells.

Autoimmune Diseases
Autoimmune diseases, such as rheumatoid arthritis, lupus, and multiple sclerosis, are characterized by the immune system mistakenly attacking the body's tissues. Chronic inflammation is a key factor in the development and progression of these diseases, and certain inflammatory foods can exacerbate symptoms and trigger flare-ups.

4.3 Role of the gut in the immune system

The gut microbiome is central to the regulation of the immune system, influencing immune development, promoting immune tolerance, and modulating inflammatory responses. Disruptions to this delicate balance can lead to immune dysregulation, chronic inflammation, and even the development of autoimmune diseases. Nurturing a healthy gut microbiome through diet and lifestyle can therefore have a profound impact on immune health and overall well-being.

Development of the Immune System

Early Immune Development: The gut microbiome is essential in shaping the development of the immune system, especially in early life. From birth, exposure to gut bacteria helps train the immune system to distinguish between harmful pathogens and harmless antigens.
Maturation of Immune Cells: Specific bacteria in the gut stimulate the maturation of various immune cells, such as T-cells and regulatory T-cells (Tregs), which are vital for maintaining immune tolerance and preventing autoimmunity.

Immune Tolerance

Preventing Overreaction: A balanced gut microbiome promotes immune tolerance by helping the body avoid overreacting to harmless substances like food proteins or its own tissues. Regulatory T-cells, which are influenced by gut bacteria, play a key role in suppressing excessive immune responses.

Dysbiosis and Autoimmunity: An imbalanced gut microbiome, or dysbiosis, can lead to inappropriate immune activation and contribute to autoimmune diseases. When harmful bacteria dominate or beneficial bacteria are depleted, the immune system may become overactive, triggering inflammatory responses.

Modulation of Inflammatory Responses

Short-Chain Fatty Acids (SCFAs): Beneficial gut bacteria, particularly Bifidobacteria and Firmicutes, produce SCFAs like butyrate, acetate, and propionate by fermenting dietary fibre. SCFAs have anti-inflammatory properties and help regulate immune responses by promoting the production of regulatory T-cells and maintaining the integrity of the intestinal lining.

Reduction of Pro-Inflammatory Cytokines: The microbiome influences the production of pro-inflammatory cytokines, such as TNF-α and IL-6, which are involved in inflammation. A healthy microbiome helps keep these cytokines in check, reducing the risk of chronic inflammation and related diseases.

Gut Barrier Function and Immune Protection

Maintaining Gut Integrity: The gut lining, or epithelial barrier, is a critical defence mechanism that prevents harmful pathogens and toxins from entering the bloodstream. The gut microbiome helps maintain this barrier by stimulating the production of mucus and tight junction proteins that keep the gut lining intact.

Leaky Gut and Immune Activation: When the gut barrier is compromised (a condition known as leaky gut), larger molecules, such as toxins or partially digested food particles, can pass into the bloodstream. This can trigger an immune response and systemic inflammation, which may contribute to autoimmune diseases.

Interaction with the Mucosal Immune System

Mucosal Immunity: The gut-associated lymphoid tissue (GALT) is a key part of the immune system located in the gut lining. The gut microbiome interacts with this immune tissue, stimulating the production of secretory IgA, an antibody that helps neutralize pathogens before they can breach the gut barrier.

Pattern Recognition: Immune cells in the gut express pattern recognition receptors (e.g., Toll-like receptors, TLRs) that recognize microbial molecules. These receptors help the immune system differentiate between pathogenic and commensal (harmless or beneficial) microbes, modulating the immune response accordingly.

Systemic Immune Effects

Gut-Brain-Immune Axis: The gut microbiome also influences systemic immunity through the gut-brain-immune axis. This communication network links gut bacteria to the brain and immune system, with the gut microbiome affecting the body's stress response, inflammation, and even the onset of certain autoimmune diseases.

Systemic Inflammation: Gut bacteria produce various metabolites that circulate through the body, influencing immune cells and inflammation beyond the gut. For example, dysbiosis can lead to the production of harmful metabolites, such as lipopolysaccharides (LPS), which can trigger systemic inflammation and immune activation.

Microbiome and Autoimmune Diseases

Microbiome Dysbiosis and Autoimmunity: In autoimmune diseases like multiple sclerosis (MS), type 1 diabetes, and rheumatoid arthritis, there is often an altered gut microbiome profile. The imbalance in gut bacteria can drive immune system dysregulation and contribute to the development or exacerbation of these conditions.

Microbial Metabolites and Immune Regulation: Certain gut bacteria can produce metabolites that directly modulate immune responses. For instance, butyrate, produced by fibre-fermenting bacteria, enhances the function of regulatory T-cells, which help suppress autoimmune responses.

Diet and the Microbiome's Role in Immunity

Fiber-Rich Diet: A diet rich in fibre feeds beneficial gut bacteria, leading to the production of SCFAs that support immune health. In contrast, diets high in processed foods and low in fiber can lead to dysbiosis and chronic inflammation.

Probiotics and Prebiotics: Introducing probiotics (beneficial bacteria) and prebiotics (fibre that feeds gut bacteria) into the diet has been shown to modulate immune function, reduce inflammation, and improve symptoms of autoimmune diseases.

Therefore, the gut microbiome plays a crucial role in regulating the immune system, influencing both local immunity in the gut and systemic immune responses throughout the body. This interaction between gut bacteria and the immune system helps maintain a balance between immune tolerance and immune activation. The control and regulation of the diet and food triggers have a huge impact on response within the immune system the body and its functions.

5. Holistic Management of Autoimmune Diseases Through Diet and Lifestyle

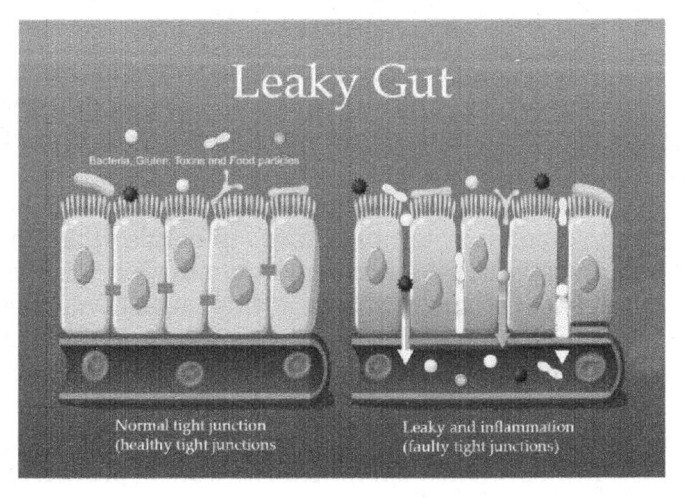

Leaky Gut

Bacteria, Gluten, Toxins and Food particles

Normal tight junction
(healthy tight junctions)

Leaky and inflammation
(faulty tight junctions)

Reducing the intake of inflammatory foods and incorporating anti-inflammatory foods into your diet can help lower inflammation levels and reduce the risk of chronic diseases. Below are some practical tips for adopting an anti-inflammatory diet:

Focus on Whole, Unprocessed Foods;
Whole, unprocessed foods are rich in essential nutrients, fibre, and antioxidants that support overall health and reduce inflammation. Prioritize the following food groups:

Fruits and vegetables: These are packed with antioxidants, vitamins, and minerals that help combat oxidative stress and inflammation. Aim for a variety of colours to ensure a wide range of nutrients.

Whole grains: Choose whole grains such as brown rice, quinoa, oats, and whole wheat, which are rich in fibre and have a lower glycaemic index compared to refined grains.

Lean proteins: opt for lean sources of protein such as poultry, fish, legumes, and plant-based proteins like tofu and tempeh.

Healthy fats: Incorporate healthy fats from sources such as olive oil, avocados, nuts, seeds, and fatty fishlike salmon and mackerel, which are high in anti-inflammatory omega-3 fatty acids.

Limit Processed Foods and Sugary Beverages

Processed foods and sugary beverages are major contributors to chronic inflammation. Minimize or eliminate these items from your diet:

Sugary drinks like soda and fruit juices with added sugars

Processed snacks and baked goods

These items often contain heightened levels of refined carbohydrates, added sugars, unhealthy fats, and artificial additives, all of which can contribute to inflammation within the body. Many processed snacks and baked goods are manufactured using refined flours, which possess a high glycaemic index and can induce a swift elevation in blood sugar levels. This surge in blood sugar can prompt the production of inflammatory compounds and foster chronic inflammation over time. In addition, these products frequently incorporate unhealthy fats, such as trans fats and specific vegetable oils rich in omega-6 fatty acids, which have been associated with heightened inflammation and oxidative stress in the body. Moreover, processed snacks and baked goods commonly feature added sugars, which can lead to spikes in blood sugar levels and stimulate the release of pro-inflammatory substances within the body. Furthermore, these items may contain artificial additives, preservatives, and flavourings, which can further contribute to inflammation and may have potential adverse effects on overall health. To sum up, processed snacks and baked goods can act as inflammatory triggers owing to their elevated levels of refined carbohydrates, added sugars, unhealthy fats, and artificial additives, all of which have the potential to induce inflammation and contribute to negative health outcomes.

Fast food and fried foods

When foods undergo the process of frying, particularly in unhealthy fats such as trans fats and vegetable oils high in omega-6 fatty acids, they generate detrimental byproducts, including advanced glycation end products (AGEs) and other toxins, which can prompt inflammation within the body. Furthermore, these types of foods often contain elevated levels of unhealthy fats, refined carbohydrates, and added sugars, all of which can contribute to a surge in blood sugar and insulin levels, thereby fostering increased inflammation. Additionally, fried and fast foods typically possess low levels of essential nutrients, including vitamins, minerals, and antioxidants, crucial for mitigating inflammation and sustaining overall health. They often contain high amounts of additives, preservatives, and artificial ingredients, further inciting inflammation. Moreover, the high caloric content of fried and fast foods can lead to weight gain and obesity, both of which are linked to chronic, low-grade inflammation within the body. In conclusion, the inflammatory triggers associated with fried foods and fast foods stem from the production of detrimental byproducts during the frying process, their high quantities of unhealthy fats, refined carbohydrates, and added sugars, their inadequate nutrient content, and their potential to induce weight gain and obesity.

Foods high in refined carbohydrates, such as white bread and pasta

Upon consumption, these carbohydrates, found in products such as white bread, pastries, and processed foods, instigate a rapid surge in blood sugar levels. This escalation prompts the body to release heightened insulin levels to regulate blood sugar. The repetitive nature of these fluctuations can lead to chronic inflammation within the body. Furthermore, refined carbohydrates boast a high glycaemic index, indicating a swift digestion and absorption process that results in rapid blood sugar increases. Consequently, the production of advanced glycation end products (AGEs) is prompted, further fuelling inflammation and oxidative stress in the body. Moreover, excessive consumption of refined carbohydrates can contribute to weight gain and obesity, conditions directly associated with heightened inflammation. Adipose tissue, or fat cells, produces pro-inflammatory substances, and an increase in body fat creates an environment conducive to chronic inflammation. Additionally, refined carbohydrates often lack essential nutrients and fibre, which are prevalent in whole, unprocessed foods such as fruits, vegetables, and whole grains. The absence of these beneficial nutrients and fibre can disrupt the balance of gut bacteria, fostering the growth of pro-inflammatory bacteria, and thus perpetuating inflammation in the body. To summarize, refined carbohydrates serve as inflammatory triggers due to their capacity to rapidly elevate blood sugar levels, promote AGEs production, contribute to weight gain and obesity, and lack essential nutrients and fibre that support a healthy internal environment.

Balance Omega-6 and Omega-3 Fatty Acids

To reduce inflammation, aim to balance your intake of omega-6 and omega-3 fatty acids. Reduce the consumption of omega-6-rich vegetable oils and processed foods, and increase your intake of omega-3-rich foods such as:
Fatty fish (e.g., salmon, sardines, mackerel)
Flaxseeds and chia seeds
Walnuts
Algal oil (a plant-based source of omega-3s)

Choose Healthy Cooking Methods

The way food is cooked can influence its inflammatory potential. Opt for healthier cooking methods, such as steaming, grilling, baking, and sautéing, rather than frying. Cooking at lower temperatures can also help reduce the formation of harmful compounds like AGEs.

Stay Hydrated

Proper hydration is essential for maintaining overall health and reducing inflammation. Water is the best choice for staying hydrated, as sugary beverages and alcohol can contribute to inflammation.

Inflammatory foods, such as refined carbohydrates, sugary beverages, trans fats, and processed meats, can contribute to chronic inflammation and increase the risk of various health conditions, including cardiovascular disease, diabetes, obesity, cancer, and autoimmune disorders. By understanding the role of diet in inflammation and making healthier food choices, individuals can reduce their risk of chronic diseases and improve overall health.

An anti-inflammatory diet emphasizes whole, unprocessed foods rich in nutrients, fibre, and antioxidants while limiting inflammatory foods that promote oxidative stress and the release of pro-inflammatory markers. By adopting an anti-inflammatory lifestyle, individuals can support their immune system, reduce inflammation, and promote long-term well-being.

While genetics play a significant role in determining susceptibility to autoimmune diseases, they do not fully explain the increasing incidence and prevalence of these disorders. Environmental triggers are now recognized as critical factors that interact with genetic predispositions to influence the onset, progression, and severity of autoimmune diseases.

Influence of Diet

Diet exerts a significant influence on the onset and regulation of autoimmune diseases. Various dietary components have been implicated in the development and management of autoimmune conditions.

Research indicates that certain foods can either trigger or alleviate inflammation, thereby directly impacting autoimmune diseases. Components such as gluten and dairy have been correlated with heightened inflammation, potentially exacerbating autoimmune disease symptoms. Conversely, a diet abundant in fruits, vegetables, and healthy fats has been associated with reduced inflammation and may aid in the management of autoimmune conditions. Moreover, specific dietary regimens, such as the Mediterranean diet or an anti-inflammatory diet, have demonstrated favourable effects on autoimmune diseases. These diets typically prioritize whole, unprocessed foods, healthy fats, and anti-inflammatory spices, which can modulate the immune system and decrease inflammation. Individuals managing autoimmune diseases are advised to collaborate with healthcare professionals, including registered dietitians or nutritionists, to devise personalized dietary plans tailored to their specific condition, food sensitivities, and nutritional requirements. Making informed dietary choices represents a crucial aspect of autoimmune disease management and overall health promotion.

5.1 Food Intolerance

Food intolerance refers to the body's inability to properly digest certain foods, which can lead to various symptoms such as bloating, diarrhoea, or stomach pain. Unlike food allergies, which trigger the immune system, food intolerances typically involve difficulty digesting specific components of food, such as lactose or gluten. This can result from enzyme deficiencies or sensitivities to certain food additives. Food intolerances can vary widely in terms of severity and can be managed through dietary adjustments and, in some cases, the use of enzyme supplements.

If not treated, intolerances can result in inflammation and an immune response. When an individual experiences an intolerance to specific foods or substances, it can potentially lead to chronic inflammation. This chronic inflammatory response occurs because of the body's immune system reacts to the perceived threat posed by the intolerances, leading to persistent inflammation.

When an individual experiences an intolerance to specific foods or substances, the body's immune system may interpret these as potential threats, triggering an inflammatory response. This response may involve the activation and release of immune cells and inflammatory mediators, leading to the onset of inflammation within the body when there has been exposure over a prolonged period.

There is substantial medical evidence supporting the notion that intolerance to certain substances can elicit an immune response. When the body perceives a particular substance as harmful, the immune system may initiate a response, leading to symptoms such as inflammation, digestive disturbances, skin ailments, or respiratory complications. This immune response serves as the body's mechanism for neutralizing the perceived threat. Common intolerances that may prompt immune responses include gluten intolerance (celiac disease), lactose intolerance, and food sensitivities to specific components. If there is a suspicion of intolerance leading to an immune response, it is imperative to seek consultation with a qualified healthcare professional for appropriate evaluation and management.

Intolerance testing has the potential to assist in the identification of specific substances that may elicit an adverse immune response in individuals. By identifying these intolerances, individuals may have the opportunity to make dietary or environmental adjustments aimed at avoiding the initiation of prolonged immune responses. This proactive approach has the potential to contribute to the prevention of sustained immune system activation and its associated complications. However, it is important to acknowledge that the efficacy of intolerance testing in averting long-term immune responses may vary based on individual circumstances and the specific intolerances identified. Seeking guidance from a qualified healthcare professional can offer personalized insights into the potential role of intolerance testing in mitigating prolonged immune responses.

As of 2023, prevalent autoimmune conditions in the UK include rheumatoid arthritis, psoriasis, multiple sclerosis, inflammatory bowel disease (encompassing ulcerative colitis and Crohn's disease), systemic lupus erythematosus, and Hashimoto's thyroiditis.

These conditions significantly impact a considerable portion of the UK population, leading to diverse effects on overall health and quality of life. It is imperative to acknowledge that the prevalence of autoimmune conditions may continue to evolve. A comprehensive understanding of these contributing factors is vital in elucidating the intricate mechanisms underlying autoimmune responses and in developing precise therapeutic interventions for autoimmune disorders.

5.2 Lifestyle Management

Managing autoimmune conditions requires careful consideration of lifestyle and dietary choices, which can significantly impact symptom management and overall well-being. Implementing the following strategies may prove beneficial:

1. Nutrition: Embracing a well-rounded, balanced diet comprising a variety of fruits, vegetables, whole grains, lean proteins, and healthy fats can aid in mitigating inflammation and supporting overall health. Furthermore, individuals with autoimmune conditions may find tailored dietary interventions, such as adhering to an anti-inflammatory diet or eliminating trigger foods, advantageous.

2. Physical Activity: Regular exercise contributes to enhanced strength, flexibility, and overall energy levels. Low-impact activities like yoga, swimming, or

walking may particularly benefit individuals with autoimmune conditions due to their gentle nature.

3. Stress Management: Given the exacerbating effects of stress on autoimmune condition symptoms, the practice of stress-reducing activities such as meditation, deep breathing exercises, or engaging in hobbies is recommended.

4. Quality Sleep: Adequate and restful sleep is crucial for supporting the immune system and promoting overall health. Establishing a consistent sleep schedule and cultivating a relaxing bedtime routine are conducive to improved sleep quality.

5. Supplementation: For certain individuals, specific dietary supplements like omega-3 fatty acids, vitamin D, or probiotics may be advantageous. Prior consultation with a healthcare provider is essential before commencing any new supplement regimen.

6. Professional Consultation: Collaboration with healthcare professionals, including physicians and nutritionists, ensures personalized recommendations and close monitoring of the effectiveness and safety of lifestyle and dietary modifications. Understanding the variability in individual responses to lifestyle and dietary adjustments underscores the importance of a tailored approach guided by healthcare expertise and supervision.

The management of autoimmune diseases is significantly influenced by nutrition, diet, and intolerances. The established connection between dietary choices, immune system function, and inflammation underscores the pivotal role of nutrition in the context of autoimmune conditions.

Additionally, specific dietary intolerances or sensitivities have the potential to exacerbate symptoms and contribute to immune system dysregulation. Therefore, a comprehensive understanding of the importance of nutrition, adherence to appropriate dietary recommendations, and the identification and management of potential intolerances are imperative in effectively addressing autoimmune diseases and advancing overall wellness.

This brings us to the role of most identified food intolerances and the foods that are anti-inflammatory to combat these. It must be noted that some individuals will be intolerant or even allergic to the inflammatory foods therefore the self-help notion must be preceded with an intolerance test.

The foods most associated with intolerances are dairy products, gluten-containing grains, nuts, shellfish, and specific fruits or vegetables. Individuals with autoimmune conditions frequently experience exacerbation of symptoms or immune system reactions upon consuming these foods. Therefore, the identification and management of intolerances to these specific foods are paramount in the comprehensive management of autoimmune diseases.

What are allergies?

Allergies, in essence, denote an immune system's reaction to a specific substance, whereas intolerance does not entail immune system involvement. In cases of allergies, the immune system identifies a harmless substance as a threat and manifests an exaggerated response, precipitating symptoms such as hives, pruritus, swelling, and in severe instances, anaphylaxis. Conversely, intolerance does not implicate the immune system but rather relates to the body's incapacity to digest or metabolize certain foods, culminating in manifestations like bloating, flatulence, or diarrhoea. While allergies can potentially be life-threatening, intolerances typically provoke less severe reactions.

5.3 Inflammatory Foods

Inflammatory foods are those that have the potential to contribute to bodily inflammation.
Examples of such foods include:
Refined sugars,
Artificial trans fats,
Vegetable oils high in omega-6 fatty acids,
Processed meats,
Artificial colours
Artificial preservatives and additives including thickeners
Excessive alcohol consumption.
These food items may exacerbate inflammatory conditions and are recommended to be either avoided or consumed in moderation, particularly for individuals with autoimmune diseases or other conditions associated with inflammation. It is advisable to seek guidance from healthcare

professionals or registered dietitians to determine the most appropriate dietary choices based on individual health requirements.

5.4 Anti-inflammatory Spices include:

1. Turmeric: Rich in curcumin, a compound known for its potent anti-inflammatory properties.

Turmeric contains a compound known as curcumin, which exhibits anti-inflammatory properties through its ability to inhibit the activity of specific enzymes and proteins involved in the inflammatory process. Furthermore, curcumin has demonstrated the capacity to reduce the production of inflammatory chemicals in the body. As a result, turmeric is frequently utilized as a natural remedy to alleviate symptoms associated with inflammatory conditions such as arthritis. Incorporating turmeric into one's diet or using turmeric supplements may contribute to the mitigation of inflammation. Nonetheless, it is advisable to consult a healthcare professional prior to commencing any new supplementation, especially if concurrent medications are being taken or if existing health conditions are present.

2. Ginger: Renowned for its anti-inflammatory and antioxidant effects.

Ginger is known for its anti-inflammatory properties, which may aid in the reduction of inflammation within the body. It contains bioactive compounds such as gingerol, believed to possess anti-inflammatory and antioxidant effects. These compounds have the potential to inhibit the production of specific inflammatory markers in the body, offering potential relief for conditions associated with inflammation, such as arthritis. Additionally, ginger may contribute to the alleviation of muscle pain and soreness, further demonstrating its potential as an anti-inflammatory agent. However, it is imperative to engage in consultation with a healthcare professional prior to utilizing ginger as a treatment for any specific health condition, in order to ascertain its safety and suitability in relation to individual health requirements.

3. Cinnamon: Contains antioxidants and exhibits anti-inflammatory properties.

Cinnamon is recognized for its anti-inflammatory properties attributed to its abundant levels of antioxidants, particularly polyphenols. These antioxidants play a crucial role in mitigating inflammation by counteracting oxidative stress and neutralizing free radicals within the body. Furthermore, cinnamon harbours compounds that are thought to impede specific inflammatory enzymes, thereby diminishing the body's inflammatory response. Consequently, the consumption of cinnamon or the use of cinnamon essential oil may contribute to the alleviation of inflammation and associated symptoms. It is imperative to note, however, that while cinnamon may offer anti-inflammatory advantages, it is not a substitute for professional medical advice and treatment. Before integrating cinnamon or any other natural remedies for inflammatory conditions, it is essential to seek guidance from a healthcare professional.

4. Cayenne pepper: Contains capsaicin, which has demonstrated inflammation-reducing properties.

Cayenne pepper contains an active compound known as capsaicin, which confers upon it anti-inflammatory properties. Capsaicin functions as a potent inhibitor of substance P, a neuropeptide pivotal in the inflammatory process. Through the reduction of substance P levels, capsaicin mitigates pain and inflammation. Furthermore, capsaicin may modulate the activity of specific immune cells, thereby augmenting its anti-inflammatory effects. Integration of cayenne pepper into the diet may offer potential benefits for managing inflammatory conditions. Nevertheless, it is paramount to seek guidance from a healthcare professional before implementing substantial dietary or lifestyle modifications, especially for individuals with underlying health concerns.

5. Cloves: Abundant in antioxidants and traditionally utilized for their anti-inflammatory effects.

Cloves contain compounds with anti-inflammatory properties, which may aid in reducing inflammation within the body. One of the active components in cloves is eugenol, a substance that has been the subject of research into its potential anti-inflammatory effects. The consumption of cloves or clove oil has been suggested as a possible approach to managing inflammation associated with conditions such as arthritis, muscle aches, and other inflammatory disorders. However, it is essential to seek guidance from a healthcare professional prior to using cloves or clove oil for medicinal purposes to ensure appropriateness and safety in relation to individual health requirements.

6. Garlic: Contains sulphur compounds with established anti-inflammatory properties.

Garlic is widely acknowledged for its potential anti-inflammatory properties due to the presence of sulphur compounds, notably allicin. These compounds have been the subject of research regarding their capacity to mitigate inflammation within the body by potentially inhibiting the activity of pro-inflammatory substances. Furthermore, the antioxidant characteristics of garlic may contribute to its anti-inflammatory effects by counteracting free radicals known to contribute to inflammation. Nevertheless, while the potential of garlic as an anti-inflammatory agent shows promise, further comprehensive research is warranted to fully elucidate its mechanisms and efficacy in this domain. As with any dietary or healthcare-related inquiry, consulting with a qualified healthcare professional is recommended for personalized guidance.

7. Black pepper: Contains piperine, which shows potential anti-inflammatory effects.

The compound piperine present in black pepper is believed to exhibit anti-inflammatory properties. It is thought to potentially suppress the expression of specific pro-inflammatory substances in the body, thus reducing inflammation. Furthermore, black pepper's substantial antioxidant content may also contribute to its anti-inflammatory effects by counteracting free radicals known to incite inflammation. While existing evidence supports the potential anti-inflammatory properties of black pepper, further research is necessary to comprehensively comprehend its mechanisms and efficacy. Seeking personalized advice from a healthcare professional is advisable for any inquiries related to dietary and health concerns.

8. Rosemary: Contains rosmarinic acid, known for its anti-inflammatory properties.

Rosemary contains compounds such as carnosic acid and rosmarinic acid, which have demonstrated anti-inflammatory properties. These compounds are believed to mitigate inflammation by inhibiting the activity of specific enzymes involved in the inflammatory process. Moreover, the antioxidants present in rosemary may help counteract free radicals and diminish oxidative stress, thereby contributing to the reduction of inflammation. Integrating rosemary into one's diet or utilizing rosemary essential oil in aromatherapy or topically may offer potential benefits in combating inflammation. Nonetheless, it is advisable to seek guidance from a healthcare professional before incorporating rosemary or any alternative remedies for managing inflammation, particularly for individuals with underlying health conditions or those taking medications.

9. Thyme: Encompasses compounds with documented anti-inflammatory effects.

Thyme contains compounds, such as rosmarinic acid and flavonoids, which exhibit anti-inflammatory properties by inhibiting specific enzymes that promote inflammation in the body. Particularly, rosmarinic acid has demonstrated the ability to mitigate inflammation and prevent the release of pro-inflammatory cytokines. Furthermore, thyme is rich in essential oils with documented anti-inflammatory and antioxidant effects. These attributes position thyme as a prospective natural remedy for attenuating inflammation, potentially benefitting individuals with inflammatory conditions. However, it is imperative to seek guidance from a healthcare professional before integrating thyme or any other natural remedies into an inflammation management regimen, particularly for individuals with preexisting health conditions or those taking medications.

10. Saffron: Contains compounds with potential anti-inflammatory properties.

Saffron contains compounds such as crocin, safranal, and crocetin, which are purported to possess anti-inflammatory properties. These compounds may inhibit the activity of specific enzymes involved in promoting inflammation within the body. Additionally, saffron is thought to modulate the immune response and reduce the production of inflammatory molecules. Nonetheless, further investigation is required to comprehensively elucidate the mechanisms through which saffron exerts its anti-inflammatory effects. Before using saffron or any other supplement for its anti-inflammatory properties, it is essential to seek guidance from a healthcare professional.

What are antioxidants and how do they help the body?

Antioxidants are molecules that can prevent, or slow down cellular damage caused by free radicals. Free radicals are unstable molecules capable of inducing oxidative stress, a process that can lead to cellular damage. Antioxidants function by donating one of their electrons to neutralize free radicals, thereby stabilizing them and reducing their potential to cause damage. This process contributes to the protection of the body from oxidative stress and may play a role in reducing the risk of chronic diseases such as heart disease, cancer, and certain neurological conditions. Antioxidants are present in a variety of foods, including fruits, vegetables, nuts, and whole grains. Consumption of a diet rich in antioxidants is associated with the support of overall health and well-being.

Integration of these spices into dietary practices may contribute to mitigating inflammation and fostering overall health.

5.5 Anti-inflammatory Fruits

1. Berries (such as strawberries, blueberries, raspberries)

Berries are acknowledged for their anti-inflammatory properties due to their high concentration of antioxidants, particularly flavonoids and anthocyanins. These bioactive compounds have demonstrated anti-inflammatory effects by reducing the levels of inflammatory markers in the body. Furthermore, the significant fibre content in berries contributes to their anti-inflammatory characteristics, supporting gut health and mitigating inflammation in the digestive system. In summary, the presence of antioxidants and fiber in berries renders them advantageous for ameliorating inflammation within the body.

2. Cherries

Cherries are known for their anti-inflammatory properties attributed to their high levels of antioxidants and specific compounds such as anthocyanins and cyanidin. These bioactive compounds have demonstrated the ability to mitigate inflammatory processes, particularly in conditions such as arthritis and gout. The consumption of cherries or cherry juice has shown promise in managing inflammation and ameliorating symptoms associated with inflammatory disorders.

3. Pineapple

Pineapples are recognized for their anti-inflammatory properties primarily owing to the presence of bromelain, an enzyme with established anti-inflammatory effects. Bromelain has demonstrated efficacy in mitigating swelling, bruising, and discomfort associated with inflammation, potentially modulating the immune response and ameliorating the severity of inflammatory conditions such as arthritis and sinusitis. Furthermore, pineapples are abundant in antioxidants, such as vitamin C, which further contribute to their potential anti-inflammatory properties.

4. Papaya

Papaya is recognized for its anti-inflammatory properties, primarily due to the presence of an enzyme called papain. Papain has demonstrated efficacy in reducing inflammation, aiding in digestion, and enhancing overall immune health. In addition to papain, papaya contains a rich array of antioxidants, including vitamins A, C, and E, which further contribute to its potential anti-inflammatory properties. Including papaya in the diet may be beneficial for combating inflammation and promoting overall well-being.

5. Watermelon

Watermelon contains a natural compound known as lycopene, which has demonstrated anti-inflammatory properties. Lycopene functions as a potent antioxidant, aiding in the neutralization of free radicals within the body that contribute to inflammation. Furthermore, watermelon is a rich source of vitamin C and other antioxidants, which also play a role in mitigating inflammation. The inclusion of watermelon in a well-rounded diet may aid in promoting overall health and eliciting an anti-inflammatory response within the body.

6. Oranges

Oranges possess anti-inflammatory properties attributed to their high levels of vitamin C and various antioxidants, such as flavonoids. These bioactive compounds contribute to attenuating inflammation by counteracting free radicals and inhibiting inflammatory pathways within the body. The incorporation of oranges into one's dietary regimen may engender an overall anti-inflammatory response while bolstering the body's inherent defence mechanisms.

Vitamin C and flavonoids help prevent inflammation through their antioxidant properties. Vitamin C is known to neutralize free radicals, which can trigger inflammation. Additionally, flavonoids have been found to inhibit the activity of certain enzymes that trigger the body's inflammatory response. As a result, the combination of these compounds helps to limit inflammation by counteracting free radicals and inhibiting specific inflammatory pathways within the body.

7. Grapefruits

Grapefruit is another fruit with high content of Vitamin C and flavonoids which play a significant role in mitigating inflammation through their antioxidant properties. Vitamin C functions in the neutralization of free radicals, which can incite inflammation. Moreover, flavonoids have demonstrated the ability to impede the activity of specific enzymes that initiate the body's inflammatory response. Consequently, the combination of these compounds effectively restricts inflammation by counteracting free radicals and inhibiting select inflammatory pathways within the body.

8. Apples

Apples are rich in quercetin, a flavonoid known for its anti-inflammatory properties. Quercetin functions by inhibiting histamine release, thereby reducing the body's inflammatory response. Furthermore, the high antioxidant content in apples, particularly vitamin C, contributes to their anti-inflammatory effects by neutralizing free radicals, which are implicated in the initiation of inflammation. Consequently, the consumption of apples is associated with the potential to effectively mitigate inflammation owing to the presence of these bioactive compounds.

What are free radicals and their role in inflammation?

It is easy to talk about free radicals but what are they exactly?

Free radicals are highly reactive atoms or molecules with unpaired electrons. They play a significant role in causing inflammation by damaging cells, proteins, and DNA through a process known as oxidative stress. This damage can trigger an inflammatory response in the body as it attempts to repair and remove the affected cells. Consequently, inflammation caused by free radicals is associated with various chronic diseases and aging processes

MEAT AND FISH

Certain categories of meat, specifically fatty fish and grass-fed beef, contain anti-inflammatory omega-3 fatty acids and other advantageous nutrients. Fatty fish varieties, such as salmon and mackerel, are abundant in omega-3s, which have demonstrated anti-inflammatory properties. Grass-fed beef also harbours elevated levels of omega-3s and antioxidants in comparison to conventionally raised beef. It is pertinent to note, however, that processed and red meats have been linked to heightened inflammation. Hence, moderation and prudent selection of healthier alternatives are essential considerations when contemplating the anti-inflammatory attributes of meat.

If the meat is not interfered with through processing and additives such as colours and preservatives, then less health issues but currently, this is seldom the case.

Chicken meat contains all essential amino acids, including leucine, isoleucine, valine, lysine, methionine, phenylalanine, threonine, tryptophan, and histidine. However, no specific amino acid is exclusively found in chicken meat.

ESSENTIAL AMINO ACIDS

The human body cannot produce nine essential amino acids on its own. These are
histidine,
isoleucine,
leucine,
lysine,
methionine,
phenylalanine,
threonine,
tryptophan, and
valine.

Therefore, it's essential to obtain these amino acids from the diet. If you opt for a vegetarian or a vegan diet, then you need to ensure that your food is also providing you with the essential amino acids that your body can only obtain from your food.

Certain categories of meat, such as fatty fish and grass-fed beef, contain anti-inflammatory omega-3 fatty acids and other beneficial nutrients. Fatty fish varieties, such as salmon and mackerel, are rich in omega-3s, which have demonstrated anti-inflammatory properties. Similarly, grass-fed beef is also high in omega-3s and antioxidants compared to conventionally raised beef.

It is important to note, however, that processed and red meats have been associated with increased inflammation. Therefore, maintaining moderation and opting for healthier alternatives are essential considerations when evaluating the anti-inflammatory properties of meat.

Fruits and vegetables typically do not provide all nine essential amino acids that the human body cannot produce on its own. However, maintaining a diverse plant-based diet incorporating legumes, quinoa, soy products, chia seeds, buckwheat, and hemp seeds can ensure the intake of all essential amino acids necessary for the body. Furthermore, strategically combining various plant-based foods throughout the day can facilitate the complete acquisition of essential amino acids.

Quinoa, soybeans, hemp seeds, chia seeds, and buckwheat are examples of grains, legumes, and seeds that provide all nine essential amino acids required by the human body. The inclusion of these foods in one's diet can facilitate the comprehensive acquisition of essential amino acids, ensuring proper nutritional intake.

Beans, such as soybeans, black beans, and kidney beans, are recognized as valuable sources of essential amino acids crucial for human health. These legumes offer a well-balanced profile of essential amino acids, thus serving as significant protein sources, particularly for individuals adhering to a vegetarian or vegan dietary regimen.

VEGAN/VEGETARIAN DIET

A vegan or vegetarian diet may lead to deficiencies in several key vitamins, potentially causing health issues. These deficiencies commonly include
vitamin B12,
vitamin D,
iron,
calcium,
omega-3 fatty acids, and
zinc.

It is imperative for individuals adhering to these dietary patterns to be mindful of ensuring sufficient intake of these nutrients through fortified foods or supplements to preserve optimal health.

Non-meat sources of vitamin D include fortified foods such as specific types of dairy and plant-based milk, orange juice, and breakfast cereals. Exposure to sunlight also stimulates the body's production of vitamin D.

In terms of calcium, non-meat sources encompass dairy products, fortified plant-based milk, tofu, almonds, and dark leafy greens such as kale and bok choy.

Non-meat sources of iron include legumes, tofu, pumpkin seeds, quinoa, and spinach.

Zinc rich non-meat sources include legumes, seeds, nuts, dairy products (or fortified plant-based dairy), and whole grains.

A non-inflammatory diet is typically characterized by a rich array of fruits and vegetables containing antioxidants and compounds known for their anti-inflammatory properties, such as vitamin C, flavonoids, and quercetin. Additionally, the inclusion of omega-3 fatty acid-rich fatty fish, grass-fed beef, and other lean meats is advantageous. Whole grains, nuts, and seeds are also integral components of an anti-inflammatory diet, along with sources of healthy fats such as olive oil and avocados. It is essential to limit the intake of processed and red meats, as well as foods high in added sugars and trans fats when striving to adhere to an anti-inflammatory dietary approach.

A well-rounded vegan diet should encompass a diverse selection of foods to meet the body's requirements for essential vitamins and amino acids. Primarily, for vitamin B12, which is predominantly found in animal-derived products, vegans can seek out fortified foods or consider B12 supplementation. Legumes, seeds, nuts, and soy products serve as essential sources of amino acids such as lysine, methionine, and tryptophan. Additionally, a varied intake of fruits, vegetables, whole grains, and fortified plant-based milk can contribute the necessary vitamins and minerals, including iron, calcium, vitamin D, and omega-3 fatty acids.

An anti-inflammatory balanced vegan diet should encompass a diverse range of nutrient-dense foods. This includes the incorporation of fruits such as berries, cherries, and oranges, as well as vegetables like leafy greens, tomatoes, and bell peppers to provide essential vitamins, minerals, and antioxidants. Whole grains such as quinoa and brown rice, along with legumes like lentils and chickpeas, are valuable sources of fibre and beneficial plant compounds. Furthermore, integrating healthy fats from sources like avocados, nuts, and seeds, and incorporating spices renowned for their anti-inflammatory properties such as turmeric and ginger can further bolster the support for an anti-inflammatory diet.

MENTAL/EMOTIONAL STRESS AND AUTOIMMUNE DISEASE TRIGGER

The relationship between mental stress and the triggering of autoimmune diseases is multifaceted and not yet fully elucidated. However, it is widely posited that persistent stress can disrupt immune system regulation, thereby heightening susceptibility to autoimmune disorders. Prolonged stress can induce the release of stress-related hormones, notably cortisol, which can impact immune function. Moreover, stress has been associated with the promotion of inflammation within the body, and chronic inflammation is frequently implicated in the onset and exacerbation of autoimmune maladies. Additionally, stress can influence the composition of the gut microbiome, which plays a pivotal role in immune modulation and has been linked to autoimmune diseases. It is important to acknowledge that while evidence suggests a correlation between stress and autoimmune diseases, complex mechanisms are still under investigation, and individual responses to stress may vary. Implementing stress management strategies such as mindfulness, relaxation techniques, and seeking social support may be beneficial for overall well-being, particularly in the context of autoimmune conditions.

Elevated levels of cortisol, commonly known as the stress hormone, can initiate and exacerbate autoimmune responses by modulating the body's immune function. In the presence of stress, cortisol is released as part of the innate fight-or-flight response. Prolonged exposure to heightened cortisol levels may suppress immune system activity, rendering the body more vulnerable to infections and compromising its capacity to modulate inflammation. Disruption of immune functionality may contribute to the onset and escalation of autoimmune disorders. Furthermore, chronic stress and elevated cortisol levels have been associated with heightened inflammation, a hallmark of several autoimmune conditions. Thus, managing stress and cortisol levels could potentially mitigate the impact of autoimmune reactions.

PHYSICAL STRESS AND TRIGGER OF AUTOIMMUNE CONDITIONS

The physical manifestation of stress can initiate the production of stress hormones, notably cortisol, which can exert a significant impact on the body's immune function. Upon perception of physical stress, the body activates the 'fight or flight' response, leading to the secretion of cortisol. Elevated cortisol levels can suppress immune system activity, rendering the body more susceptible to infections and impairing its ability to regulate inflammation. This disruption of immune functionality may contribute to the onset and exacerbation of autoimmune disorders. Furthermore, chronic physical stress and heightened cortisol levels have been linked to increased inflammation, a critical factor in numerous autoimmune conditions. Consequently, the management of physical stress and cortisol levels may hold the potential to ameliorate the initiation of autoimmune responses within the body.

A good example is the reported cases of Alopecia start after a significant emotional or physical shock to the body.

Alopecia can be triggered by a significant shock or traumatic event, a phenomenon known as telogen effluvium. This condition arises when a sudden or stressful event disrupts the normal hair growth cycle, causing many hair follicles to simultaneously enter the resting (telogen) phase. This, in turn, leads to excessive shedding of hair and noticeable hair loss. While the precise mechanisms linking shock or trauma to alopecia are not fully elucidated, it is widely believed that the body's response to stress can impact the hair growth cycle, resulting in temporary hair loss.

COLLAGEN PEPTIDE HYPE

The relationship between collagen peptides and gut health is well-established. Collagen peptides, due to their unique amino acid profile, have been shown to contribute to the maintenance and repair of the gut lining. This can have a positive impact on overall gut health and function. Furthermore, the presence of specific amino acids in collagen peptides, such as glycine, proline, and glutamine, may aid in supporting the integrity of the gut lining and regulating stomach acid secretion. These factors are crucial for the balance of gut microbiota and the overall well-being of the digestive system.

5.6 What is a leaky gut?

Leaky gut, medically referred to as increased intestinal permeability, is a condition characterized by the heightened permeability of the small intestine lining. This increased permeability can result in the passage of undigested food particles, toxins, and potentially harmful substances into the bloodstream. It is widely believed to be linked to various health complications, as the immune system may mount a response to these substances, leading to inflammation and other associated issues.

Increased intestinal permeability, commonly known as leaky gut, has gained prominence in the realm of health and wellness. The term refers to a condition in which the intestinal barrier becomes compromised, allowing undigested food particles, toxins, and harmful substances to pass into the bloodstream. This heightened permeability has been associated with a range of health concerns, as the immune system may react to these substances, triggering inflammation and potentially contributing to various health complications. The intestinal lining serves as a critical barrier, facilitating the absorption of nutrients while preventing the entry of harmful substances into the bloodstream. When the integrity of this barrier is compromised, as is the case with leaky gut, the selective permeability is disrupted. While the precise causes of leaky gut remain the subject of ongoing research, several factors have been implicated in its development. These may include chronic stress, poor dietary habits, imbalances in gut microbiota, excessive alcohol consumption, prolonged use of nonsteroidal anti-inflammatory drugs (NSAIDs), and certain medical conditions such as celiac disease and Crohn's disease. Genetic predisposition is also believed to play a role in susceptibility to developing leaky gut. The impact of a leaky gut on overall health is a topic of ongoing exploration. While the concept was initially met with scepticism in conventional medical circles, emerging evidence has shed light on its potential role in various health conditions. It is important to note that while leaky gut has been associated with certain health issues, it does not imply causation, and further research is needed to establish definitive links. One of the primary concerns associated with a leaky gut is its potential impact on the immune system. The intestines house a significant portion of the body's immune cells and play a pivotal role in immune function. When the intestinal barrier is compromised, the immune system may become activated in response to the influx of harmful substances from the gut into the bloodstream. This immune response can lead to chronic inflammation, which has been linked to a range of health conditions, including autoimmune disorders, allergies, and inflammatory bowel diseases. Furthermore, leaky gut has been hypothesized to influence the development of certain chronic diseases. Research suggests that increased intestinal permeability may be associated with conditions such as irritable bowel syndrome (IBS), inflammatory bowel disease (IBD), celiac disease, and food allergies. While the exact nature of these associations is still being elucidated, the potential role of leaky gut in contributing to the pathogenesis of these conditions is an area of active investigation. In addition to immune-related and gastrointestinal issues, a leaky gut has been suggested to impact other aspects of health, including mental well-being. The gut-brain axis, which refers to the bidirectional communication between the gut and the brain, has gained attention in the context of various neurological and psychiatric conditions. Some research suggests that the disruption of the intestinal barrier and subsequent immune activation may play a role in conditions such as depression, anxiety, and neurodegenerative diseases. Addressing leaky gut and its potential impact on health involves a multifaceted approach. Strategies aimed at promoting gut health, such as adhering to a balanced diet rich in fibre and nutrients, supporting a healthy gut microbiota through the consumption of probiotics and fermented foods, managing stress, and minimizing exposure to potential gut irritants, may play a role in maintaining intestinal barrier integrity. Additionally, identifying and addressing underlying medical conditions and minimizing the use of medications that may contribute to intestinal damage are important considerations in the management of a leaky gut. In conclusion, leaky gut represents a complex and multifaceted area of study within the realm of health and wellness. While the concept of increased intestinal permeability and its potential health implications continue to be explored, it is evident that the integrity of the intestinal barrier is of paramount importance. Understanding the factors that contribute to a leaky gut, its potential impact on immune function, gastrointestinal health, and overall well-being, and implementing strategies to support gut health are essential components of ongoing research and clinical practice. As our understanding of leaky gut evolves, it holds the potential to inform novel approaches to promoting holistic health and well-being.

To repair a leaky gut, it is recommended to consume certain foods. These include bone broth, which contains amino acids that support gut health, as well as fermented foods like kimchi and sauerkraut, known to improve gut flora. Additionally, foods rich in fibre such as fruits, vegetables, and whole grains can aid in the restoration of a healthy gut lining. Consumption of foods high in omega-3 fatty acids like salmon and chia seeds can also contribute to reducing inflammation in the gut and support its healing process.

Foods abundant in dietary fibre, encompassing fruits, vegetables, and whole grains, can bolster gut health by fostering the growth of common bacteria and serving as a substrate for intestinal cell metabolism. Additionally, probiotic-rich foods like yogurt, kefir, and fermented vegetables can aid in reestablishing a harmonious gut microbiota composition.

THE SPLEEN AND ROLE IN IMMUNE REGULATION

The connection between specific dietary constituents and the spleen resides in the spleen's pivotal role in immunological surveillance and haematological processes. The spleen functions in the removal of defective erythrocytes and contributes to combatting select bacterial infections. Foods that bolster overall immune competence and haematological integrity, such as those rich in antioxidants, vitamins, and minerals, may indirectly support spleen function. Nevertheless, it is imperative to underscore that while certain dietary components can fortify general gut health and immune function, singular foods cannot directly target or rectify splenic function.

The spleen is an essential organ that plays a pivotal role in regulating the immune system and mitigating autoimmunity. As the largest secondary lymphoid organ, the spleen serves as a filter for the blood and is integral to both innate and adaptive immune responses. Its strategic positioning and unique structure enable it to carry out several vital functions crucial for sustaining immune equilibrium and averting the onset of autoimmune conditions. At the forefront of its functions, the spleen acts as a blood filter, removing aged or impaired red blood cells, platelets, and pathogens. This process is instrumental in upholding the general well-being and functionality of the blood, while also preventing the accumulation of potentially detrimental substances in the circulatory system. Moreover, the spleen acts as a reservoir for immune cells, including lymphocytes and macrophages, and serves as a site for instigating immune responses against blood-borne pathogens. In the realm of adaptive immunity, the spleen assumes a critical role in eliciting specific immune responses to antigens. It serves as a site for the activation and proliferation of B cells, which are responsible for generating antibodies against foreign pathogens. Additionally, the spleen is involved in presenting antigens to T cells, thereby facilitating the development of cellular immune responses.

These processes are indispensable for efficiently eliminating pathogens and establishing immunological memory, which confers enduring protection against reinfection. Furthermore, the spleen is integral to the reticuloendothelial system, responsible for clearing immune complexes and apoptotic cells. This function is crucial in averting the accumulation of self-antigens and the onset of autoimmune responses by ensuring the effective removal of cellular debris and potentially immunogenic material. Hence, the spleen contributes to the preservation of self-tolerance and the prevention of autoimmunity. In the context of autoimmunity, the spleen plays a pivotal role in regulating immune responses to self-antigens.

It serves as a site for inducing peripheral tolerance mechanisms, such as the elimination of autoreactive lymphocytes and the generation of regulatory T cells. These processes are indispensable in preventing the activation of self-reactive immune cells and the development of autoimmune diseases. Moreover, the spleen partakes in clearing circulating immune complexes and regulating inflammatory responses, critical for maintaining immune equilibrium and preventing the progression of autoimmune pathologies.

In summary, the spleen assumes a central role in regulating the immune system and averting autoimmunity through its involvement in blood filtration, immune cell trafficking, antigen presentation, and peripheral tolerance mechanisms. Its distinctive anatomical and functional attributes render it an indispensable organ for sustaining immune homeostasis and preventing autoimmune diseases. A comprehensive understanding of the spleen's role in immune regulation is crucial for devising innovative therapeutic strategies for treating autoimmune disorders and enhancing immune responses against infectious agents.

Certain vitamins and peptides have been recognized for their potential to support the function of the spleen.

These include:
Vitamin D:
Acknowledged for its immunomodulatory properties, vitamin D plays a role in regulating immune responses and contributing to overall immune function, which can indirectly impact the spleen.

Vitamin C:
Vitamin C, a potent antioxidant, aids the immune system by safeguarding cells from oxidative stress and facilitating the absorption of iron, crucial for red blood cell production in the spleen.

Thymosin alpha-1:
This peptide has been the subject of research due to its immunomodulatory characteristics and it's potential to enhance immune function, including its impact on the spleen's role in immune responses. While these vitamins and peptides are associated with bolstering immune function, it is imperative to seek guidance from a healthcare professional before considering the use of supplements to ensure their suitability for individual health requirements.

Thymosin alpha-1 is not naturally found in dietary sources but is produced synthetically for medical and research purposes. Bioactive peptides from protein hydrolysates: Certain bioactive peptides derived from protein hydrolysates have been investigated for their potential immunomodulatory effects, which may indirectly impact the function of the spleen. These peptides can be obtained from various dietary protein sources such as milk, eggs, fish, and certain grains through processes like enzymatic hydrolysis. While research on the direct dietary sources of peptides that specifically target the spleen is ongoing, incorporating a balanced and varied protein-rich diet may support overall immune function, including potential benefits for spleen health.

ZINC AND ITS ROLE IN THE IMMUNE SYSTEM

Zinc plays a crucial role in maintaining a healthy immune system. It is involved in numerous aspects of immune function, including:

1. Enzyme function:

Zinc is essential for the proper functioning of over 300 enzymes involved in various biochemical reactions in the body, including those related to immune system function.

2. Immune cell development and function:

Zinc is vital for the development and function of immune cells, including neutrophils, natural killer cells, and T-lymphocytes. These cells play a key role in the body's defence against pathogens.

3. Inflammatory response:

Zinc helps regulate the immune system's inflammatory response. It helps modulate the production of cytokines, which are signalling molecules involved in the immune response to infections and injuries.

4. Antioxidant activity:
Zinc acts as an antioxidant, helping to protect cells from oxidative stress and supporting overall immune function. Adequate zinc intake is important for maintaining a robust immune system, and a zinc deficiency can impair immune function, leading to an increased susceptibility to infections.

Good dietary sources of zinc include meat, shellfish, legumes, seeds, nuts, dairy products, and whole grains. Additionally, zinc supplements may be recommended for individuals at risk of deficiency, but it's important to consult with a healthcare professional before starting any supplementation.

5.7 Deficiencies in dietary vitamins and minerals

Zinc plays a crucial role in maintaining a healthy immune system. It is involved in numerous aspects of immune function, including: 1. Enzyme function: Zinc is essential for the proper functioning of over 300 enzymes involved in various biochemical reactions in the body, including those related to immune system function. 2. Immune cell development and function: Zinc is vital for the development and function of immune cells, including neutrophils, natural killer cells, and T-lymphocytes. These cells play a key role in the body's defence against pathogens. 3. Inflammatory response: Zinc helps regulate the immune system's inflammatory response.

It helps modulate the production of cytokines, which are signalling molecules involved in the immune response to infections and injuries. 4. Antioxidant activity: Zinc acts as an antioxidant, helping to protect cells from oxidative stress and supporting overall immune function. Adequate zinc intake is important for maintaining a robust immune system, and a zinc deficiency can impair immune function, leading to an increased susceptibility to infections. Good dietary sources of zinc include meat, shellfish, legumes, seeds, nuts, dairy products, and whole grains. Additionally, zinc supplements may be recommended for individuals at risk of deficiency, but it's important to consult with a healthcare professional before starting any supplementation.

Deficiencies in vitamins and minerals can potentially contribute to the development of autoimmune diseases or dysregulation in the immune system. Adequate intake of essential vitamins and minerals is crucial for maintaining a well-functioning immune system and promoting immune tolerance, which helps prevent the immune system from attacking the body's tissues.

For example, vitamin D deficiency has been linked to an increased risk of autoimmune diseases such as multiple sclerosis, rheumatoid arthritis, and type 1 diabetes. Vitamin D plays a role in immune regulation and deficiency may lead to immune dysregulation. Similarly, deficiencies in other nutrients such as vitamin C, vitamin A, vitamin E, zinc, selenium, and omega-3 fatty acids have been associated with altered immune function and increased susceptibility to infections and inflammatory conditions, which may contribute to autoimmune disease development or immune dysregulation.

It's important to maintain a balanced and nutritious diet to ensure adequate intake of essential vitamins and minerals for optimal immune function and overall health. If there are concerns about nutritional deficiencies or their potential impact on immune health, consulting with a healthcare professional or a registered dietitian is recommended for personalized guidance. Too many people try to self-help without consulting a professional and they end up overconsuming vitamins and minerals that can also have a detrimental side effect.

Conclusion

Autoimmune diseases are complex disorders influenced by both genetic and environmental factors. While genetic predisposition plays a significant role, environmental triggers such as infections, diet, pollutants, toxins, stress, and lifestyle factors are critical in the development and progression of these diseases. Understanding these triggers and their mechanisms of action can help inform strategies for prevention, early diagnosis, and targeted treatment of autoimmune diseases. By reducing exposure to environmental risk factors and supporting immune health through lifestyle modifications, individuals may be able to lower their risk of developing autoimmune conditions or improve their quality of life if they are already affected.

While genetics play a significant role in determining susceptibility to autoimmune diseases, they do not fully explain the increasing incidence and prevalence of these disorders. Environmental triggers are now recognized as critical factors that interact with genetic predispositions to influence the onset, progression, and severity of autoimmune diseases.

Understanding the environmental triggers of autoimmune diseases can help elucidate how and why these conditions develop, leading to more effective strategies for prevention, diagnosis, and treatment. My aim for this book was to discuss and explore the range of environmental triggers that contribute to autoimmune disease, including infections, diet, pollutants, toxins, stress, lifestyle factors, and more.

Additionally, I wanted to create an understanding and awareness of the mechanisms by which these environmental factors interact with the immune system to promote autoimmune processes and how they contribute to specific autoimmune diseases.

While genetic predisposition is important, it does not fully explain the onset of autoimmune diseases. Many individuals with a genetic predisposition never develop the disease, while others without a strong genetic background do. This suggests that environmental factors play a crucial role in triggering autoimmunity in genetically susceptible individuals.

Auto immune Conditions have been extensively studied for their physical impacts, but their effects on mental health are often less understood or overlooked. However, it is now well-established that autoimmune diseases can significantly affect mental health, leading to psychological distress, mood disorders, cognitive dysfunction, and a decline in overall quality of life.

In researching and writing Unmasking Autoimmune Disease, I have delved into the various ways autoimmune diseases can impact mental health, examining the biological, psychological, and social mechanisms underlying these effects. I have also discussed how the physical burden of autoimmune diseases interacts with emotional and cognitive aspects, and how managing mental health is crucial for improving outcomes in patients with autoimmune conditions. I do hope that this information can help you and your loved ones have a better understanding of autoimmune diseases and how to have some degree of self-management through diet and lifestyle.

For information and advice, please go to

www.asafoundation.org.uk

info@asafoundation.org.uk

REFERENCES

1. Çehreli R. Moleculer nutritional immunology and cancer. J. Oncol. Sci. 2018;4:40–46. doi: 10.1016/j.jons.2018.02.002. [CrossRef] [Google Scholar]

2. Platt A.M. Immunity in the Gut. Viral Gastroenteritis. 2017;351:1329–1333. [Google Scholar]

3. Lerner A., Matthias T. Changes in intestinal tight junction permeability associated with industrial food additives explain the rising incidence of autoimmune disease. Autoimmune. Rev. 2015;14:479–489. doi: 10.1016/j.autrev.2015.01.009. [PubMed] [CrossRef] [Google Scholar]

4. Venter C., Eyerich S., Sarin T., Klatt K.C. Nutrition and the immune system: A complicated tango. Nutrients. 2020;12:818. doi: 10.3390/nu12030818. [PMC free article] [PubMed] [CrossRef] [Google Scholar]

5. Rose N.R. Prediction and prevention of autoimmune disease in the 21st century: A review and preview. Am. J. Epidemiol. 2016;183:403–406. doi: 10.1093/aje/kwv292. [PubMed] [CrossRef] [Google Scholar]

6. De Luca F., Shoenfeld Y. The microbiome in autoimmune diseases. Clin. Exp. Immunol. 2019;195:74–85. doi: 10.1111/cei.13158. [PMC free article] [PubMed] [CrossRef] [Google Scholar]

7. Okada H., Kuhn C., Feillet H., Bach J.-F. The 'hygiene hypothesis' for autoimmune and allergic diseases: An update. Clin. Exp. Immunol.

2010;160:1–9. doi: 10.1111/j.1365-2249.2010.04139.x. [PMC free article] [PubMed] [CrossRef] [Google Scholar]

8. Selmi C. The worldwide gradient of autoimmune conditions. Autoimmun. Rev. 2010;9:A247–A250. doi: 10.1016/j.autrev.2010.02.004. [PubMed] [CrossRef] [Google Scholar]

9. Brady B.D.M. Autoimmune disease: A modern epidemic? Molecular mimicry, the hygiene hypothesis, stealth infections, and other examples of disconnect between medical research and the practice of clinical medicine. N. Engl. J. Med. 2014;347:911–920. doi: 10.4236/ojra.2013.31007. [CrossRef] [Google Scholar]

10. Fatoye F., Gebrye T., Svenson L.W. Real-world incidence and prevalence of systemic lupus erythematosus in Alberta, Canada. Rheumatol. Int. 2018;38:1721–1726. doi: 10.1007/s00296-018-4091-4. [PMC free article] [PubMed] [CrossRef] [Google Scholar]

11. Fasano A., Shea-Donohue T. Mechanisms of disease: The role of intestinal barrier function in the pathogenesis of gastrointestinal autoimmune diseases. Nat. Clin. Pract. Gastroenterol. Hepatol. 2005;2:416–422. doi: 10.1038/ncpgasthep0259. [PubMed] [CrossRef] [Google Scholar]

12. Buckland G., Agudo A., Travier N., Huerta J.M., Cirera L., Tormo M.-J., Navarro C., Chirlaque M.D., Moreno-Iribas C., Ardanaz E., et al. Adherence to the Mediterranean diet reduces mortality in the Spanish cohort of the European Prospective Investigation into Cancer and Nutrition (EPIC-Spain)

Br. J. Nutr. 2011;106:1581–1591. doi: 10.1017/S0007114511002078. [PubMed] [CrossRef] [Google Scholar]

13. Naska A., Trichopoulou A. Back to the future: The Mediterranean diet paradigm. Nutr. Metab. Cardiovasc. Dis. 2014;24:216–219. doi: 10.1016/j.numecd.2013.11.007. [PubMed] [CrossRef] [Google Scholar]

14. Monteiro C.A., Cannon G., Levy R.B., Moubarac J.C., Louzada M.L.C., Rauber F., Khandpur N., Cediel G., Neri D., Martinez-Steele E., et al. Ultra-processed foods: What they are and how to identify them. Public Health Nutr. 2019;22:936–941. doi: 10.1017/S1368980018003762. [PMC free article] [PubMed] [CrossRef] [Google Scholar]

15. Varlamov O. Western-style diet, sex steroids and metabolism. Biochim. Biophys. Acta -Mol. Basis Dis. 2017;1863:1147–1155. doi: 10.1016/j.bbadis.2016.05.025. [PubMed] [CrossRef] [Google Scholar]

16. Gioia C., Lucchino B., Tarsitano M.G., Iannuccelli C., Di Franco M. Dietary habits and nutrition in rheumatoid arthritis: Can diet influence disease development and clinical manifestations? Nutrients. 2020;12:1456. doi: 10.3390/nu12051456. [PMC free article] [PubMed] [CrossRef] [Google Scholar]

17. Desai M.S., Seekatz A.M., Koropatkin N.M., Kamada N., Hickey C.A., Wolter M., Pudlo N.A., Kitamoto S., Terrapon N., Muller A., et al. A dietary fiber-deprived gut microbiota degrades the colonic mucus barrier and enhances pathogen susceptibility. Cell. 2016;167:1339–1353. doi:

10.1016/j.cell.2016.10.043. [PMC free article] [PubMed] [CrossRef] [Google Scholar]

18. Maione F., Cappellano G., Bellan M., Raineri D., Chiocchetti A. Chicken-or-egg question: Which came first, extracellular vesicles or autoimmune diseases? J. Leukoc. Biol. 2020;108:601–616. doi: 10.1002/JLB.3MR0120-232R. [PMC free article] [PubMed] [CrossRef] [Google Scholar]

19. Munger K.L., Levin L.I., Hollis B.W., Howard N.S., Ascherio A. Serum 25-hydroxyvitamin D levels and risk of multiple sclerosis. JAMA. 2006;296:2832–2838. doi: 10.1001/jama.296.23.2832. [PubMed] [CrossRef] [Google Scholar]

20. Christ A., Lauterbach M., Latz E. Western diet and the immune system: An inflammatory connection. Immunity. 2019;51:794–811. doi: 10.1016/j.immuni.2019.09.020. [PubMed] [CrossRef] [Google Scholar]

21. Huang S., Rutkowsky J.M., Snodgrass R.G., Ono-Moore K.D., Schneider D.A., Newman J.W., Adams S.H., Hwang D.H. Saturated fatty acids activate TLR-mediated proinflammatory signaling pathways. J. Lipid Res. 2012;53:2002–2013. doi: 10.1194/jlr.D029546. [PMC free article] [PubMed] [CrossRef] [Google Scholar]

22. Timmermans S., Bogie J.F.J., Vanmierlo T., Lütjohann D., Stinissen P., Hellings N., Hendriks J.J.A. High fat diet exacerbates neuroinflammation in an animal model of multiple sclerosis by activation of the renin angiotensin system. J. Neuroimmune Pharmacol. 2014;9:209–217. doi: 10.1007/s11481-013-9502-4. [PubMed] [CrossRef] [Google Scholar]

23. Katz Sand I. The role of diet in multiple sclerosis: Mechanistic connections and current evidence. Curr. Nutr. Rep. 2018;7:150–160. doi: 10.1007/s13668-018-0236-z. [PMC free article] [PubMed] [CrossRef] [Google Scholar]

24. Hagen K.B., Byfuglien M.G., Falzon L., Olsen S.U., Smedslund G. Dietary interventions for rheumatoid arthritis. Cochrane Database Syst. Rev. 2009 doi: 10.1002/14651858.CD006400.pub2. [PubMed] [CrossRef] [Google Scholar]

25. Cena H., Calder P.C. Defining a healthy diet: Evidence for the role of contemporary dietary patterns in health and disease. Nutrients. 2020;12:334. doi: 10.3390/nu12020334. [PMC free article] [PubMed] [CrossRef] [Google Scholar]

26. Martínez-González M.A., Sánchez-Villegas A. The emerging role of Mediterranean diets in cardiovascular epidemiology: Monounsaturated fats, olive oil, red wine or the whole pattern? Eur. J. Epidemiol. 2004;19:9–13. doi: 10.1023/B:EJEP.0000013351.60227.7b. [PubMed] [CrossRef] [Google Scholar]

27. Forsyth C., Kouvari M., D'Cunha N.M., Georgousopoulou E.N., Panagiotakos D.B., Mellor D.D., Kellett J., Naumovski N. The effects of the Mediterranean diet on rheumatoid arthritis prevention and treatment: A systematic review of human prospective studies. Rheumatol. Int. 2018;38:737–747. doi: 10.1007/s00296-017-3912-1. [PubMed] [CrossRef] [Google Scholar]

28. Davis C., Bryan J., Hodgson J., Murphy K. Definition of the mediterranean diet: A literature review. Nutrients. 2015;7:9139–9153. doi:

10.3390/nu7115459. [PMC free article] [PubMed] [CrossRef] [Google Scholar]

29. Calder P.C. Omega-3 fatty acids and inflammatory processes: From molecules to man. Biochem. Soc. Trans. 2017;45:1105–1115. doi: 10.1042/BST20160474. [PubMed] [CrossRef] [Google Scholar]

30. Nelson J., Sjöblom H., Gjertsson I., Ulven S.M., Lindqvist H.M., Bärebring L. Do interventions with diet or dietary supplements reduce the disease activity score in rheumatoid arthritis? A systematic review of randomized controlled trials. Nutrients. 2020;12:2991. doi: 10.3390/nu12102991. [PMC free article] [PubMed] [CrossRef] [Google Scholar]

31. Simopoulos A.P. The importance of the omega-6/omega-3 fatty acid ratio in cardiovascular disease and other chronic diseases. Exp. Biol. Med. 2008;233:674–688. doi: 10.3181/0711-MR-311. [PubMed] [CrossRef] [Google Scholar]

32. Anderson B.M., Ma D.W.L. Are all n-3 polyunsaturated fatty acids created equal? Lipids Health Dis. 2009;8:1–20. doi: 10.1186/1476-511X-8-33. [PMC free article] [PubMed] [CrossRef] [Google Scholar]

33. Statovci D., Aguilera M., MacSharry J., Melgar S. The impact of western diet and nutrients on the microbiota and immune response at mucosal interfaces. Front. Immunol. 2017;8:838. doi: 10.3389/fimmu.2017.00838. [PMC free article] [PubMed] [CrossRef] [Google Scholar]

34. Atarashi K., Tanoue T., Oshima K., Suda W., Nagano Y., Nishikawa H., Fukuda S., Saito T., Narushima S., Hase K., et al. Treg induction by a

rationally selected mixture of Clostridia strains from the human microbiota. Nature. 2013;500:232–236. doi: 10.1038/nature12331. [PubMed] [CrossRef] [Google Scholar]

35. Arpaia N., Campbell C., Fan X., Dikiy S., van der Veeken J., de Roos P., Liu H., Cross J.R., Pfeffer K., Coffer P.J., et al. Metabolites produced by commensal bacteria promote peripheral regulatory T-cell generation. Nature. 2013;504:451–455. doi: 10.1038/nature12726. [PMC free article] [PubMed] [CrossRef] [Google Scholar]

36. Strate L.L., Keeley B.R., Cao Y., Wu K., Giovannucci E.L., Chan A.T. Western dietary pattern increases, and prudent dietary pattern decreases, risk of incident diverticulitis in a prospective cohort study. Gastroenterology. 2017;152:1023–1030. doi: 10.1053/j.gastro.2016.12.038. [PMC free article] [PubMed] [CrossRef] [Google Scholar]

37. Bennett E., Peters S.A.E., Woodward M. Sex differences in macronutrient intake and adherence to dietary recommendations: Findings from the UK Biobank. BMJ Open. 2018;8:e020017. doi: 10.1136/bmjopen-2017-020017. [PMC free article] [PubMed] [CrossRef] [Google Scholar]

38. Zaccardelli A., Friedlander H.M., Ford J.A., Sparks J.A. Potential of lifestyle changes for reducing the risk of developing rheumatoid arthritis: Is an ounce of prevention worth a pound of cure? Clin. Ther. 2019;41:1323–1345. doi: 10.1016/j.clinthera.2019.04.021. [PMC free article] [PubMed] [CrossRef] [Google Scholar]

39. Sharma M., Rao M., Jacob S., Jacob C.K. Validation of 24-hour dietary recall: A study in

hemodialysis patients. J. Ren. Nutr. 1998;8:199–202. doi: 10.1016/S1051-2276(98)90018-8. [PubMed] [CrossRef] [Google Scholar]

40. Steinemann N., Grize L., Ziesemer K., Kauf P., Probst-Hensch N., Brombach C. Relative validation of a food frequency questionnaire to estimate food intake in an adult population. Food Nutr. Res. 2017;61:1305193. doi: 10.1080/16546628.2017.1305193. [PMC free article] [PubMed] [CrossRef] [Google Scholar]

41. Fatihah F., Ng B.K., Hazwanie H., Karim Norimah A., Shanita S.N., Ruzita A.T., Poh B.K. Development and validation of a food frequency questionnaire for dietary intake assessment among multi-ethnic primary school-aged children. Singap. Med. J. 2015;56:687–694. doi: 10.11622/smedj.2015190. [PMC free article] [PubMed] [CrossRef] [Google Scholar]

42. Affret A., El Fatouhi D., Dow C., Correia E., Boutron-Ruault M.C., Fagherazzi G. Relative validity and reproducibility of a new 44-item diet and food frequency questionnaire among adults: Online assessment. J. Med. Internet Res. 2018;20:e9113. [PMC free article] [PubMed] [Google Scholar]

43. García-Conesa M.T., Philippou E., Pafilas C., Massaro M., Quarta S., Andrade V., Jorge R., Chervenkov M., Ivanova T., Dimitrova D., et al. Exploring the validity of the 14-item mediterranean diet adherence screener (Medas): A cross-national study in seven european countries around the mediterranean region. Nutrients. 2020;12:2960. doi: 10.3390/nu12102960. [PMC free article] [PubMed] [CrossRef] [Google Scholar]

44. Turconi G., Celsa M., Rezzani C., Biino G., Sartirana M.A., Roggi C. Reliability of a dietary questionnaire on food habits, eating behaviour and nutritional knowledge of adolescents. Eur. J. Clin. Nutr. 2003;57:753–763. doi: 10.1038/sj.ejcn.1601607. [PubMed] [CrossRef] [Google Scholar]

45. Goldbohm R.A., Van't Veer P., Van den Brandt P.A., Van't Hof M.A., Brants H.A.M., Sturmans F., Hermus R.J.J. Reproducibility of a food frequency questionnaire and stability of dietary habits determined from five annually repeated measurements. Eur. J. Clin. Nutr. 1995;49:420–429. [PubMed] [Google Scholar]

46. Riboli E., Kaaks R. The EPIC project: Rationale and study design. European Prospective Investigation into Cancer and Nutrition. Int. J. Epidemiol. 1997;26:S6–S14. doi: 10.1093/ije/26.suppl_1.S6. [PubMed] [CrossRef] [Google Scholar]

47. Slimani N., Deharveng G., Unwin I., Southgate D.A.T., Vignat J., Skeie G., Salvini S., Parpinel M., Møller A., Ireland J., et al. The EPIC nutrient database project (ENDB): A first attempt to standardize nutrient databases across the 10 European countries participating in the EPIC study. Eur. J. Clin. Nutr. 2007;61:1037–1056. doi: 10.1038/sj.ejcn.1602679. [PubMed] [CrossRef] [Google Scholar]

48. de Pablo P., Romaguera D., Fisk H.L., Calder P.C., Quirke A.-M., Cartwright A.J., Panico S., Mattiello A., Gavrila D., Navarro C., et al. High erythrocyte levels of the n-6 polyunsaturated fatty

acid linoleic acid are associated with lower risk of subsequent rheumatoid arthritis in a southern European nested case—control study. Ann. Rheum. Dis. 2018;77:981–987. doi: 10.1136/annrheumdis-2017-212274. [PubMed] [CrossRef] [Google Scholar]

49. Vagnani S., Tani C., Carli L., Querci F., Della Rossa A., D'Ascanio A., Ermini I., Ceroti M., Caini S., Palli D., et al. Nutritional assessment in patients with systemic lupus erythematosus and systemic sclerosis. Arthritis Rheumatol. 2014;66:S1061–S1062. doi: 10.1002/art.38914. [CrossRef] [Google Scholar]

50. Keeble M., Adams J., Sacks G., Vanderlee L., White C.M., Hammond D., Burgoine T. Use of online food delivery services to order food prepared away-from-home and associated sociodemographic characteristics: A cross-sectional, multi-country analysis. Int. J. Environ. Res. Public Health. 2020;17:5190. doi: 10.3390/ijerph17145190. [PMC free article] [PubMed] [CrossRef] [Google Scholar]

51. Salgado E., Bes-Rastrollo M., de Irala J., Carmona L., Gómez-Reino J.J. High sodium intake is associated with self-reported rheumatoid arthritis: A cross sectional and case control analysis within the SUN cohort. Medicine. 2015;94:e924. doi: 10.1097/MD.0000000000000924. [PMC free article] [PubMed] [CrossRef] [Google Scholar]

52. McGuire S., Todd J.E., Mancino L., Lin B., Jessica E. The impact of food away from home on adult diet quality. USDA-ERS Econ. Res. Rep. Pap. Adv. Nutr. 2011;2:442–443. doi: 10.3945/an.111.000679. [PMC free article] [PubMed] [CrossRef] [Google Scholar]

53. Demmler K.M., Klasen S., Nzuma J.M., Qaim M. Supermarket purchase contributes to nutrition-related non-communicable diseases in urban Kenya. PLoS ONE. 2017;12:e0185148. doi: 10.1371/journal.pone.0185148. [PMC free article] [PubMed] [CrossRef] [Google Scholar]

54. Heidemann C., Schulze M.B., Franco O.H., van Dam R.M., Mantzoros C.S., Hu F.B. Dietary patterns and risk of mortality from cardiovascular disease, cancer, and all causes in a prospective cohort of women. Circulation. 2008;118:230–237. doi: 10.1161/CIRCULATIONAHA.108.771881. [PMC free article] [PubMed] [CrossRef] [Google Scholar]

55. Moore L.V., Diez Roux A.V., Nettleton J.A., Jacobs D.R., Franco M. Fast-food consumption, diet quality, and neighborhood exposure to fast food: The multi-ethnic study of atherosclerosis. Am. J. Epidemiol. 2009;170:29–36. doi: 10.1093/aje/kwp090. [PMC free article] [PubMed] [CrossRef] [Google Scholar]

56. Ramezankhani A., Hosseini-Esfahani F., Mirmiran P., Azizi F., Hadaegh F. The association of priori and posteriori dietary patterns with the risk of incident hypertension: Tehran Lipid and Glucose Study. J. Transl. Med. 2021;19:1–11. doi: 10.1186/s12967-021-02704-w. [PMC free article] [PubMed] [CrossRef] [Google Scholar]

57. Newby P.K., Tucker K.L. Empirically derived eating patterns using factor or cluster analysis: A review. Nutr. Rev. 2004;62:177–203. doi: 10.1111/j.1753-4887.2004.tb00040.x. [PubMed] [CrossRef] [Google Scholar]

58. Hu F.B., Rimm E., Smith-Warner S.A., Feskanich D., Stampfer M.J., Ascherio A., Sampson L., Willett W.C. Reproducibility and validity of dietary patterns assessed with a food-frequency questionnaire. Am. J. Clin. Nutr. 1999;69:243–249. doi: 10.1093/ajcn/69.2.243. [PubMed] [CrossRef] [Google Scholar]

59. Panagiotakos D.B., Pitsavos C., Stefanadis C. a-priori and a-posterior dietary pattern analyses have similar estimating and discriminating ability in predicting 5-y incidence of cardiovascular disease: Methodological issues in nutrition assessment. J. Food Sci. 2009;74:H218–H224. doi: 10.1111/j.1750-3841.2009.01268.x. [PubMed] [CrossRef] [Google Scholar]

60. Leermakers E.T.M., van den Hooven E.H., Franco O.H., Jaddoe V.W.V., Moll H.A., Kiefte-de Jong J.C., Voortman T. A priori and a posteriori derived dietary patterns in infancy and cardiometabolic health in childhood: The role of body composition. Clin. Nutr. 2018;37:1589–1595. doi: 10.1016/j.clnu.2017.08.010. [PubMed] [CrossRef] [Google Scholar]

61. Khaled K., Hundley V., Almilaji O., Koeppen M., Tsofliou F. A priori and a posteriori dietary patterns in women of childbearing age in the UK. Nutrients. 2020;12:2921. doi: 10.3390/nu12102921. [PMC free article] [PubMed] [CrossRef] [Google Scholar]

62. Serra-Majem L., Ribas L., Ngo J., Ortega R.M., García A., Pérez-Rodrigo C., Aranceta J. Food, youth and the Mediterranean diet in Spain. Development of

KIDMED, Mediterranean Diet Quality Index in children and adolescents. Public Health Nutr. 2004;7:931–935. doi: 10.1079/PHN2004556. [PubMed] [CrossRef] [Google Scholar]

63. Sofi F., Macchi C., Abbate R., Gensini G.F., Casini A. Mediterranean diet and health status: An updated meta-analysis and a proposal for a literature-based adherence score. Public Health Nutr. 2013;17:2769–2782. doi: 10.1017/S1368980013003169. [PMC free article] [PubMed] [CrossRef] [Google Scholar]

64. Monteagudo C., Mariscal-Arcas M., Rivas A., Lorenzo-Tovar M.L., Tur J.A., Olea-Serrano F. Proposal of a Mediterranean diet serving score. PLoS ONE. 2015;10:e0128594. doi: 10.1371/journal.pone.0128594. [PMC free article] [PubMed] [CrossRef] [Google Scholar]

65. Hodge A., Bassett J. What can we learn from dietary pattern analysis? Public Health Nutr. 2016;19:191–194. doi: 10.1017/S1368980015003730. [PMC free article] [PubMed] [CrossRef] [Google Scholar]

66. Trichopoulou A., Costacou T., Bamia C., Trichopoulos D. Adherence to a Mediterranean diet and survival in a Greek population. N. Engl. J. Med. 2003;348:2599–2608. doi: 10.1056/NEJMoa025039. [PubMed] [CrossRef] [Google Scholar]

67. Solans M., Benavente Y., Saez M., Agudo A., Naudin S., Hosnijeh F.S., Noh H., Freisling H., Ferrari P., Besson C., et al. Adherence to the Mediterranean diet and lymphoma risk in the European prospective investigation into cancer and

nutrition. Int. J. Cancer. 2019;145:122–131. doi: 10.1002/ijc.32091. [PubMed] [CrossRef] [Google Scholar]

68. Shannon O.M., Stephan B.C.M., Granic A., Lentjes M., Hayat S., Mulligan A., Brayne C., Khaw K.-T., Bundy R., Aldred S., et al. Mediterranean diet adherence and cognitive function in older UK adults: The European Prospective Investigation into Cancer and Nutrition-Norfolk (EPIC-Norfolk) Study. Am. J. Clin. Nutr. 2019;110:938–948. doi: 10.1093/ajcn/nqz114. [PubMed] [CrossRef] [Google Scholar]

69. Trichopoulou A., Orfanos P., Norat T., Bueno-de-Mesquita B., Ocké M.C., Peeters P.H.M., van der Schouw Y.T., Boeing H., Hoffmann K., Boffetta P., et al. Modified Mediterranean diet and survival: EPIC-elderly prospective cohort study. BMJ. 2005;330:991–995. doi: 10.1136/bmj.38415.644155.8F. [PMC free article] [PubMed] [CrossRef] [Google Scholar]

70. Sofi F., Dinu M., Pagliai G., Marcucci R., Casini A. Validation of a literature-based adherence score to Mediterranean diet: The MEDI-LITE score. Int. J. Food Sci. Nutr. 2017;68:757–762. doi: 10.1080/09637486.2017.1287884. [PubMed] [CrossRef] [Google Scholar]

71. Shakersain B., Santoni G., Larsson S.C., Faxén-Irving G., Fastbom J., Fratiglioni L., Xu W. Prudent diet may attenuate the adverse effects of Western diet on cognitive decline. Alzheimer's Dement. 2016;12:100–109. doi: 10.1016/j.jalz.2015.08.002. [PubMed] [CrossRef] [Google Scholar]

72. Cunnane S.C. Origins and evolution of the Western diet: Implications of iodine and seafood intakes for the human brain. Am. J. Clin. Nutr. 2005;82:483. doi: 10.1093/ajcn/82.2.483. [PubMed] [CrossRef] [Google Scholar]

73. Bach-Faig A., Berry E.M., Lairon D., Reguant J., Trichopoulou A., Dernini S., Medina F.X., Battino M., Belahsen R., Miranda G., et al. Mediterranean diet pyramid today. Science and cultural updates. Public Health Nutr. 2011;14:2274–2284. doi: 10.1017/S1368980011002515. [PubMed] [CrossRef] [Google Scholar]

role of anti oxidants in autoimmune disease
References

1. Casciaro M., di Salvo E., Pace E., Ventura-Spagnolo E., Navarra M., Gangemi S. Chlorinative Stress in Age-Related Diseases: A Literature Review. Immun. Ageing. 2017;14:1–7. doi: 10.1186/s12979-017-0104-5. [PMC free article] [PubMed] [CrossRef] [Google Scholar]

2. Wang Y., Li S., Li C. Perspectives of New Advances in the Pathogenesis of Vitiligo: From Oxidative Stress to Autoimmunity. Med. Sci. Monit. Int. Med. J. Exp. Clin. Res. 2019;25:1017. doi: 10.12659/MSM.914898. [PMC free article] [PubMed] [CrossRef] [Google Scholar]

3. Ruggeri R.M., Vicchio T.M., Cristani M., Certo R., Caccamo D., Alibrandi A., Giovinazzo S., Saija A., Campennì A., Trimarchi F., et al. Oxidative Stress and Advanced Glycation End Products in Hashimoto's Thyroiditis. Thyroid. 2016;26:504–511. doi:

10.1089/thy.2015.0592. [PubMed] [CrossRef] [Google Scholar]

4. Aryaeian N., Shahram F., Mahmoudi M., Tavakoli H., Yousefi B., Arablou T., Karegar S.J. The Effect of Ginger Supplementation on Some Immunity and Inflammation Intermediate Genes Expression in Patients with Active Rheumatoid Arthritis. Gene. 2019;698:179–185. doi: 10.1016/j.gene.2019.01.048. [PubMed] [CrossRef] [Google Scholar]

5. Vaccaro M., Bagnato G., Cristani M., Borgia F., Spatari G., Tigano V., Saja A., Guarneri F., Cannavò S.P., Gangemi S. Oxidation Products Are Increased in Patients Affected by Non-Segmental Generalized Vitiligo. Arch. Dermatol. Res. 2017;309:485–490. doi: 10.1007/s00403-017-1746-z. [PubMed] [CrossRef] [Google Scholar]

6. Cannavò S.P., Riso G., Casciaro M., di Salvo E., Gangemi S. Oxidative Stress Involvement in Psoriasis: A Systematic Review. Free Radic. Res. 2019;53:829–840. doi: 10.1080/10715762.2019.1648800. [PubMed] [CrossRef] [Google Scholar]

7. Carr A.C., Maggini S. Vitamin C and Immune Function. Nutrients. 2017;9. doi: 10.3390/nu9111211. [PMC free article] [PubMed] [CrossRef] [Google Scholar]

8. Martel J., Ojcius D.M., Ko Y.-F., Ke P.-Y., Wu C.-Y., Peng H.-H., Young J.D. Hormetic Effects of Phytochemicals on Health and Longevity. Trends Endocrinol. Metab. 2019;30:335–346. doi: 10.1016/j.tem.2019.04.001. [PubMed] [CrossRef] [Google Scholar]

9. Martucci M., Ostan R., Biondi F., Bellavista E., Fabbri C., Bertarelli C., Salvioli S., Capri M., Franceschi C., Santoro A. Mediterranean Diet and Inflammaging within the Hormesis Paradigm. Nutr. Rev. 2017;75:442–455. doi: 10.1093/nutrit/nux013. [PMC free article] [PubMed] [CrossRef] [Google Scholar]

10. Kumar M., Kaur V., Kumar S., Kaur S. Phytoconstituents as Apoptosis Inducing Agents: Strategy to Combat Cancer. Cytotechnology. 2016;68:531–563. doi: 10.1007/s10616-015-9897-2. [PMC free article] [PubMed] [CrossRef] [Google Scholar]

11. Kalra E.K. Nutraceutical-Definition and Introduction. Aaps Pharmsci. 2003;5:27–28. doi: 10.1208/ps050325. [PMC free article] [PubMed] [CrossRef] [Google Scholar]

12. Nasri H., Baradaran A., Shirzad H., Rafieian-Kopaei M. New Concepts in Nutraceuticals as Alternative for Pharmaceuticals. Int. J. Prev. Med. 2014;5:1487–1499. [PMC free article] [PubMed] [Google Scholar]

13. Télessy I.G. The Role of Functional Food Security in Global Health. Elsevier; Amsterdam, The Netherlands: 2019. Nutraceuticals; pp. 409–421. [Google Scholar]

14. European Nutraceutical Association | LinkedIn. [(accessed on 29 January 2021)]; Available online: https://it.linkedin.com/company/european-nutraceutical-association

15. Aronson J.K. Defining 'Nutraceuticals': Neither Nutritious nor Pharmaceutical. Br. J. Clin.

Pharm. 2017;83:8–19. doi: 10.1111/bcp.12935. [PMC free article] [PubMed] [CrossRef] [Google Scholar]

16. Caraffa A.L., Varvara G., Spinas E., Kritas S.K., Lessiani G., Ronconi G., Saggini A., Antinolfi P., Frydas I., de Tommaso Morrison M.C., et al. Is Vitamin E an Anti-Allergic Compound? J. Biol. Regul. Homeost. Agents. 2016;30:11–15. [PubMed] [Google Scholar]

17. Choi S.M., Lim D.S., Kim M.K., Yoon S., Kacew S., Kim H.S., Lee B.-M. Inhibition of Di(2-Ethylhexyl) Phthalate (DEHP)-Induced Endocrine Disruption by Co-Treatment of Vitamins C and E and Their Mechanism of Action. J. Toxicol. Env. Health A. 2018;81:748–760. doi: 10.1080/15287394.2018.1473262. [PubMed] [CrossRef] [Google Scholar]

18. Edge R., Truscott T.G. Singlet Oxygen and Free Radical Reactions of Retinoids and Carotenoids—A Review. Antioxidants. 2018:7. doi: 10.3390/antiox7010005. [PMC free article] [PubMed] [CrossRef] [Google Scholar]

19. Murdaca G., Tonacci A., Negrini S., Greco M., Borro M., Puppo F., Gangemi S. Emerging Role of Vitamin D in Autoimmune Diseases: An Update on Evidence and Therapeutic Implications. Autoimmun. Rev. 2019;18:102350. doi: 10.1016/j.autrev.2019.102350. [PubMed] [CrossRef] [Google Scholar]

20. Sintov A.C., Yarmolinsky L., Dahan A., Ben-Shabat S. Pharmacological Effects of Vitamin D and Its Analogs: Recent Developments. Drug Discov. Today. 2014;19:1769–1774. doi:

10.1016/j.drudis.2014.06.008. [PubMed] [CrossRef] [Google Scholar]

21. Tang L., Fang W., Lin J., Li J., Wu W., Xu J. Vitamin D Protects Human Melanocytes against Oxidative Damage by Activation of Wnt/β-Catenin Signaling. Lab. Investig. 2018;98:1527–1537. doi: 10.1038/s41374-018-0126-4. [PubMed] [CrossRef] [Google Scholar]

22. Illescas-Montes R., Melguizo-Rodríguez L., Ruiz C., Costela-Ruiz V.J. Vitamin D and Autoimmune Diseases. Life Sci. 2019;233:116744. doi: 10.1016/j.lfs.2019.116744. [PubMed] [CrossRef] [Google Scholar]

23. Panche A.N., Diwan A.D., Chandra S.R. Flavonoids: An Overview. J. Nutr. Sci. 2016:5. doi: 10.1017/jns.2016.41. [PMC free article] [PubMed] [CrossRef] [Google Scholar]

24. Rengasamy K.R.R., Khan H., Gowrishankar S., Lagoa R.J.L., Mahomoodally F.M., Khan Z., Suroowan S., Tewari D., Zengin G., Hassan S.T.S., et al. The Role of Flavonoids in Autoimmune Diseases: Therapeutic Updates. Pharmacol. Ther. 2019;194:107–131. doi: 10.1016/j.pharmthera.2018.09.009. [PubMed] [CrossRef] [Google Scholar]

25. Tuñón M.J., García-Mediavilla M.V., Sánchez-Campos S., González-Gallego J. Potential of Flavonoids as Anti-Inflammatory Agents: Modulation of pro-Inflammatory Gene Expression and Signal Transduction Pathways. Curr. Drug Metab. 2009;10:256–271. doi: 10.2174/138920009787846369. [PubMed] [CrossRef] [Google Scholar]

26. Ribeiro D., Freitas M., Lima J.L.F.C., Fernandes E. Proinflammatory Pathways: The Modulation by Flavonoids. Med. Res. Rev. 2015;35:877–936. doi: 10.1002/med.21347. [PubMed] [CrossRef] [Google Scholar]

27. Wold L.E., Muralikrishnan D., Albano C.B., Norby F.L., Ebadi M., Ren J. Insulin-like Growth Factor I (IGF-1) Supplementation Prevents Diabetesinduced Alterations in Coenzymes Q 9 and Q 10. Acta Diabetol. 2003;40:85–90. doi: 10.1007/s005920300010. [PubMed] [CrossRef] [Google Scholar]

28. Lee B.J., Tseng Y.F., Yen C.H., Lin P.T. Effects of Coenzyme Q10 Supplementation (300 Mg/Day) on Antioxidation and Anti-Inflammation in Coronary Artery Disease Patients during Statins Therapy: A Randomized, Placebo-Controlled Trial. Nutr. J. 2013;12:142. doi: 10.1186/1475-2891-12-142. [PMC free article] [PubMed] [CrossRef] [Google Scholar]

29. Albano C.B., Muralikrishnan D., Ebadi M. Distribution of Coenzyme Q Homologues in Brain. Neurochem. Res. 2002;27:359–368. doi: 10.1023/A:1015591628503. [PubMed] [CrossRef] [Google Scholar]

30. Battino M., Gorini A., Villa R.F., Genova M.L., Bovina C., Sassi S., Littarru G.P., Lenaz G. Coenzyme Q Content in Synaptic and Non-Synaptic Mitochondria from Different Brain Regions in the Ageing Rat. Mech. Ageing Dev. 1995;78:173–187. doi: 10.1016/0047-6374(94)01535-T. [PubMed] [CrossRef] [Google Scholar]

31. Rauscher F.M., Sanders R.A., Watkins J.B. Effects of Coenzyme Q10 Treatment on Antioxidant

Pathways in Normal and Streptozotocin-Induced Diabetic Rats. J. Biochem. Mol. Toxicol. 2001;15:41–46. doi: 10.1002/1099-0461(2001)15:1<41::AID-JBT5>3.0.CO;2-Z. [PubMed] [CrossRef] [Google Scholar]

32. Liu Y., Alookaran J.J., Rhoads J.M. Probiotics in Autoimmune and Inflammatory Disorders. Nutrients. 2018;10:1537. doi: 10.3390/nu10101537. [PMC free article] [PubMed] [CrossRef] [Google Scholar]

33. Ishizaki A., Bi X., Nguyen L.V., Matsuda K., Pham H.V., Phan C.T.T., Khu D.T.K., Ichimura H. Effects of Short-Term Probiotic Ingestion on Immune Profiles and Microbial Translocation among HIV-1-Infected Vietnamese Children. Int. J. Mol. Sci. 2017:18. doi: 10.3390/ijms18102185. [PMC free article] [PubMed] [CrossRef] [Google Scholar]

34. Mohammed A.T., Khattab M., Ahmed A.M., Turk T., Sakr N., Khalil A.M., Abdelhalim M., Sawaf B., Hirayama K., Huy N.T. The Therapeutic Effect of Probiotics on Rheumatoid Arthritis: A Systematic Review and Meta-Analysis of Randomized Control Trials. Clin. Rheumatol. 2017;36:2697–2707. doi: 10.1007/s10067-017-3814-3. [PubMed] [CrossRef] [Google Scholar]

35. Vitaliti G., Pavone P., Guglielmo F., Spataro G., Falsaperla R. The Immunomodulatory Effect of Probiotics beyond Atopy: An Update. J. Asthma. 2014;51:320–332. doi: 10.3109/02770903.2013.862259. [PubMed] [CrossRef] [Google Scholar]

36. Choi H., Cho S.Y., Pak H.J., Kim Y., Choi J.Y., Lee Y.J., Gong B.H., Kang Y.S., Han T., Choi G., et al.

NPCARE: Database of Natural Products and Fractional Extracts for Cancer Regulation. J. Cheminform. 2017;9:2. doi: 10.1186/s13321-016-0188-5. [PMC free article] [PubMed] [CrossRef] [Google Scholar]

37. Petrovska B.B., Cekovska S. Extracts from the History and Medical Properties of Garlic. Pharmacogn. Rev. 2010;4:106. doi: 10.4103/0973-7847.65321. [PMC free article] [PubMed] [CrossRef] [Google Scholar]

38. Cellini L., Campli E.D., Masulli M., Bartolomeo S.D., Allocati N. Inhibition of Helicobacter Pylori by Garlic Extract (Allium Sativum) FEMS Immunol. Med. Microbiol. 1996;13:273–277. doi: 10.1111/j.1574-695X.1996.tb00251.x. [PubMed] [CrossRef] [Google Scholar]

39. Goncagul G., Ayaz E. Antimicrobial Effect of Garlic (Allium Sativum) Recent Pat. Antiinfect. Drug Discov. 2010;5:91–93. doi: 10.2174/157489110790112536. [PubMed] [CrossRef] [Google Scholar]

40. Sajem A.L., Gosai K. Traditional Use of Medicinal Plants by the Jaintia Tribes in North Cachar Hills District of Assam, Northeast India. J. Ethnobiol. Ethnomed. 2006;2:33. doi: 10.1186/1746-4269-2-33. [PMC free article] [PubMed] [CrossRef] [Google Scholar]

41. Majumder M., Debnath S., Gajbhiye R.L., Saikia R., Gogoi B., Samanta S.K., Das D.K., Biswas K., Jaisankar P., Mukhopadhyay R. Ricinus Communis L. Fruit Extract Inhibits Migration/Invasion, Induces Apoptosis in Breast

Cancer Cells and Arrests Tumor Progression in Vivo. Sci. Rep. 2019;9 doi: 10.1038/s41598-019-50769-x. [PMC free article] [PubMed] [CrossRef] [Google Scholar]

42. Yin H., Fretté X.C., Christensen L.P., Grevsen K. Chitosan Oligosaccharides Promote the Content of Polyphenols in Greek Oregano (Origanum Vulgare Ssp. Hirtum) J. Agric. Food Chem. 2012;60:136–143. doi: 10.1021/jf204376j. [PubMed] [CrossRef] [Google Scholar]

43. Esen G., Azaz A.D., Kurkcuoglu M., Baser K.H.C., Tinmaz A. Essential Oil and Antimicrobial Activity of Wild and Cultivated Origanum Vulgare L. Subsp. Hirtum (Link) Letswaart from the Marmara Region, Turkey. [(accessed on 24 November 2020)];Flavour Fragr. J. 2007 doi: 10.1002/ffj.1808. Available online: https://onlinelibrary.wiley.com/doi/10.1002/ffj.1808 [CrossRef] [Google Scholar]

44. Bright J.J. Curcumin and Autoimmune Disease. Adv. Exp. Med. Biol. 2007;595:425–451. doi: 10.1007/978-0-387-46401-5_19. [PubMed] [CrossRef] [Google Scholar]

45. Fernández-Moriano C., Gómez-Serranillos M.P., Crespo A. Antioxidant Potential of Lichen Species and Their Secondary Metabolites. A Systematic Review. Pharm. Biol. 2016;54:1–17. doi: 10.3109/13880209.2014.1003354. [PubMed] [CrossRef] [Google Scholar]

46. Rodriguez C., Mayo J.C., Sainz R.M., Antolín I., Herrera F., Martín V., Reiter R.J. Regulation of Antioxidant Enzymes: A Significant Role for Melatonin. J. Pineal Res. 2004;36:1–9. doi:

10.1046/j.1600-079X.2003.00092.x. [PubMed] [CrossRef] [Google Scholar]

47. Reiter R.J., Mayo J.C., Tan D.-X., Sainz R.M., Alatorre-Jimenez M., Qin L. Melatonin as an Antioxidant: Under Promises but over Delivers. J. Pineal Res. 2016;61:253–278. doi: 10.1111/jpi.12360. [PubMed] [CrossRef] [Google Scholar]

48. Liang M., Wang Z., Li H., Cai L., Pan J., He H., Wu Q., Tang Y., Ma J., Yang L. L-Arginine Induces Antioxidant Response to Prevent Oxidative Stress via Stimulation of Glutathione Synthesis and Activation of Nrf2 Pathway. Food Chem. Toxicol. 2018;115:315–328. doi: 10.1016/j.fct.2018.03.029. [PubMed] [CrossRef] [Google Scholar]

49. Li X., Bi X., Wang S., Zhang Z., Li F., Zhao A.Z. Therapeutic Potential of ω-3 Polyunsaturated Fatty Acids in Human Autoimmune Diseases. Front. Immunol. 2019;10:2241. doi: 10.3389/fimmu.2019.02241. [PMC free article] [PubMed] [CrossRef] [Google Scholar]

50. Avery J., Hoffmann P. Selenium, Selenoproteins, and Immunity. Nutrients. 2018;10:1203. doi: 10.3390/nu10091203. [PMC free article] [PubMed] [CrossRef] [Google Scholar]

51. Wichman J., Winther K.H., Bonnema S.J., Hegedüs L. Selenium Supplementation Significantly Reduces Thyroid Autoantibody Levels in Patients with Chronic Autoimmune Thyroiditis: A Systematic Review and Meta-Analysis. Thyroid. 2016;26:1681–1692. doi: 10.1089/thy.2016.0256. [PubMed] [CrossRef] [Google Scholar]

52. Sanna A., Firinu D., Zavattari P., Valera P. Zinc Status and Autoimmunity: A Systematic Review and

Meta-Analysis. Nutrients. 2018:10. doi: 10.3390/nu10010068. [PMC free article] [PubMed] [CrossRef] [Google Scholar]

53. Mirtaheri E., Pourghassem Gargari B., Kolahi S., Dehghan P., Asghari-Jafarabadi M., Hajalilou M., Shakiba Novin Z., Mesgari Abbasi M. Effects of Alpha-Lipoic Acid Supplementation on Inflammatory Biomarkers and Matrix Metalloproteinase-3 in Rheumatoid Arthritis Patients. J. Am. Coll. Nutr. 2015;34:310–317. doi: 10.1080/07315724.2014.910740. [PubMed] [CrossRef] [Google Scholar]

54. Scaramuzza A., Giani E., Redaelli F., Ungheri S., Macedoni M., Giudici V., Bosetti A., Ferrari M., Zuccotti G.V. Alpha-Lipoic Acid and Antioxidant Diet Help to Improve Endothelial Dysfunction in Adolescents with Type 1 Diabetes: A Pilot Trial. J. Diabetes Res. 2015;2015:474561. doi: 10.1155/2015/474561. [PMC free article] [PubMed] [CrossRef] [Google Scholar]

55. Fayh A.P.T., Krause M., Rodrigues-Krause J., Ribeiro J.L., Ribeiro J.P., Friedman R., Moreira J.C.F., Reischak-Oliveira A. Effects of L-Arginine Supplementation on Blood Flow, Oxidative Stress Status and Exercise Responses in Young Adults with Uncomplicated Type I Diabetes. Eur. J. Nutr. 2013;52:975–983. doi: 10.1007/s00394-012-0404-7. [PubMed] [CrossRef] [Google Scholar]

56. Abdollahzad H., Aghdashi M.A., Jafarabadi M.A., Alipour B. Effects of Coenzyme Q10 Supplementation on Inflammatory Cytokines (TNF-α, IL-6) and Oxidative Stress in Rheumatoid Arthritis Patients: A Randomized Controlled Trial. Arch. Med.

Res. 2015;46:527–533. doi: 10.1016/j.arcmed.2015.08.006. [PubMed] [CrossRef] [Google Scholar]

57. Sanoobar M., Eghtesadi S., Azimi A., Khalili M., Khodadadi B., Jazayeri S., Gohari M.R., Aryaeian N. Coenzyme Q10 Supplementation Ameliorates Inflammatory Markers in Patients with Multiple Sclerosis: A Double Blind, Placebo, Controlled Randomized Clinical Trial. Nutr. Neurosci. 2015;18:169–176. doi: 10.1179/1476830513Y.0000000106. [PubMed] [CrossRef] [Google Scholar]

58. Sanoobar M., Dehghan P., Khalili M., Azimi A., Seifar F. Coenzyme Q10 as a Treatment for Fatigue and Depression in Multiple Sclerosis Patients: A Double Blind Randomized Clinical Trial. Nutr. Neurosci. 2016;19:138–143. doi: 10.1179/1476830515Y.0000000002. [PubMed] [CrossRef] [Google Scholar]

59. Brauner H., Luthje P., Grunler J., Ekberg N.R., Dallner G., Brismar K., Brauner A. Markers of Innate Immune Activity in Patients with Type 1 and Type 2 Diabetes Mellitus and the Effect of the Anti-Oxidant Coenzyme Q10 on Inflammatory Activity. Clin. Exp. Immunol. 2014;177:478–482. doi: 10.1111/cei.12316. [PMC free article] [PubMed] [CrossRef] [Google Scholar]

60. Vasiljevic D., Veselinovic M., Jovanovic M., Jeremic N., Arsic A., Vucic V., Lucic-Tomic A., Zivanovic S., Djuric D., Jakovljevic V. Evaluation of the Effects of Different Supplementation on Oxidative Status in Patients with Rheumatoid Arthritis. Clin. Rheumatol. 2016;35:1909–1915. doi:

10.1007/s10067-016-3168-2. [PubMed] [CrossRef] [Google Scholar]

61. Arriens C., Hynan L.S., Lerman R.H., Karp D.R., Mohan C. Placebo-Controlled Randomized Clinical Trial of Fish Oil's Impact on Fatigue, Quality of Life, and Disease Activity in Systemic Lupus Erythematosus. Nutr. J. 2015;14:82. doi: 10.1186/s12937-015-0068-2. [PMC free article] [PubMed] [CrossRef] [Google Scholar]

62. Miller E., Mrowicka M., Malinowska K., Kedziora J., Majsterek I. The Effects of Whole-Body Cryotherapy and Melatonin Supplementation on Total Antioxidative Status and Some Antioxidative Enzymes in Multiple Sclerosis Patients. Pol. Merkur. Lek. Organ Pol. Tow. Lek. 2011;31:150–153. [PubMed] [Google Scholar]

63. Adamczyk-Sowa M., Sowa P., Mucha S., Zostawa J., Mazur B., Owczarek M., Pierzchała K. Changes in Serum Ceruloplasmin Levels Based on Immunomodulatory Treatments and Melatonin Supplementation in Multiple Sclerosis Patients. Med. Sci. Monit. Int. Med. J. Exp. Clin. Res. 2016;22:2484. doi: 10.12659/MSM.895702. [PMC free article] [PubMed] [CrossRef] [Google Scholar]

64. Vaghef-Mehrabany E., Homayouni-Rad A., Alipour B., Sharif S.-K., Vaghef-Mehrabany L., Alipour-Ajiry S. Effects of Probiotic Supplementation on Oxidative Stress Indices in Women with Rheumatoid Arthritis: A Randomized Double-Blind Clinical Trial. J. Am. Coll. Nutr. 2016;35:291–299. doi: 10.1080/07315724.2014.959208. [PubMed] [CrossRef] [Google Scholar]

65. Kouchaki E., Tamtaji O.R., Salami M., Bahmani F., Kakhaki R.D., Akbari E., Tajabadi-Ebrahimi M., Jafari P., Asemi Z. Clinical and Metabolic Response to Probiotic Supplementation in Patients with Multiple Sclerosis: A Randomized, Double-Blind, Placebo-Controlled Trial. Clin. Nutr. 2017;36:1245–1249. doi: 10.1016/j.clnu.2016.08.015. [PubMed] [CrossRef] [Google Scholar]

66. Helli B., Mowla K., Mohammadshahi M., Jalali M.T. Effect of Sesamin Supplementation on Cardiovascular Risk Factors in Women with Rheumatoid Arthritis. J. Am. Coll. Nutr. 2016;35:300–307. doi: 10.1080/07315724.2015.1005198. [PubMed] [CrossRef] [Google Scholar]

67. Nemes-Nagy E., Szőcs-Molnár T., Dunca I., Balogh-Sămărghiţan V., Hobai Ş., Morar R., Pusta D.L., Crăciun E.C. Effect of a Dietary Supplement Containing Blueberry and Sea Buckthorn Concentrate on Antioxidant Capacity in Type 1 Diabetic Children. Acta Physiol. Hung. 2008;95:383–393. doi: 10.1556/APhysiol.95.2008.4.5. [PubMed] [CrossRef] [Google Scholar]

68. Tam L.S., Li E.K., Leung V.Y., Griffith J.F., Benzie I.F., Lim P.L., Whitney B., Lee V.W., Lee K.K., Thomas G.N. Effects of Vitamins C and E on Oxidative Stress Markers and Endothelial Function in Patients with Systemic Lupus Erythematosus: A Double Blind, Placebo Controlled Pilot Study. J. Rheumatol. 2005;32:275–282. [PubMed] [Google Scholar]

69. Kouchaki E., Afarini M., Abolhassani J., Mirhosseini N., Bahmani F., Masoud S.A., Asemi Z.

High-Dose ω-3 Fatty Acid plus Vitamin D3 Supplementation Affects Clinical Symptoms and Metabolic Status of Patients with Multiple Sclerosis: A Randomized Controlled Clinical Trial. J. Nutr. 2018;148:1380–1386. doi: 10.1093/jn/nxy116. [PubMed] [CrossRef] [Google Scholar]

70. Jain S.K., Krueger K.S., McVie R., Jaramillo J.J., Palmer M., Smith T. Relationship of Blood Thromboxane-B2 (TxB2) with Lipid Peroxides and Effect of Vitamin E and Placebo Supplementation on TxB2 and Lipid Peroxide Levels in Type 1 Diabetic Patients. Diabetes Care. 1998;21:1511–1516. doi: 10.2337/diacare.21.9.1511. [PubMed] [CrossRef] [Google Scholar]

71. Şardaş S., Yilmaz M., Öztok U., Çakir N., Karakaya A.E. Assessment of DNA Strand Breakage by Comet Assay in Diabetic Patients and the Role of Antioxidant Supplementation. Mutat. Res. Genet. Toxicol. Environ. Mutagenesis. 2001;490:123–129. doi: 10.1016/S1383-5718(00)00157-1. [PubMed] [CrossRef] [Google Scholar]

72. Giannini C., Lombardo F., Curro F., Pomilio M., Bucciarelli T., Chiarelli F., Mohn A. Effects of High-dose Vitamin E Supplementation on Oxidative Stress and Microalbuminuria in Young Adult Patients with Childhood Onset Type 1 Diabetes Mellitus. Diabetes/Metab. Res. Rev. 2007;23:539–546. doi: 10.1002/dmrr.717. [PubMed] [CrossRef] [Google Scholar]

73. Gupta S., Sharma T.K., Kaushik G.G., Shekhawat V.P. Vitamin E Supplementation May Ameliorate Oxidative Stress in Type 1 Diabetes

Mellitus Patients. Clin. Lab. 2011;57:379. [PubMed] [Google Scholar]

74. Cazeau R.M., Huang H., Bauer J.A., Hoffman R.P. Effect of Vitamins C and E on Endothelial Function in Type 1 Diabetes Mellitus. J. Diabetes Res. 2016;2016:3271293. doi: 10.1155/2016/3271293. [PMC free article] [PubMed] [CrossRef] [Google Scholar]

75. Hossein Nia B., Khorram S., Rezazadeh H., Safaiyan A., Tarighat-Esfanjani A. The Effects of Natural Clinoptilolite and Nano-Sized Clinoptilolite Supplementation on Glucose Levels and Oxidative Stress in Rats With Type 1 Diabetes. Can. J. Diabetes. 2018;42:31–35. doi: 10.1016/j.jcjd.2017.01.010. [PubMed] [CrossRef] [Google Scholar]

76. Shivanna N., Naika M., Khanum F., Kaul V.K. Antioxidant, Anti-Diabetic and Renal Protective Properties of Stevia Rebaudiana. J. Diabetes Complicat. 2013;27:103–113. doi: 10.1016/j.jdiacomp.2012.10.001. [PubMed] [CrossRef] [Google Scholar]

77. Wang W., Wang C., Ding X.Q., Pan Y., Gu T.T., Wang M.X., Liu Y.L., Wang F.M., Wang S.J., Kong L.D. Quercetin and Allopurinol Reduce Liver Thioredoxin-Interacting Protein to Alleviate Inflammation and Lipid Accumulation in Diabetic Rats. Br. J. Pharmacol. 2013;169:1352–1371. doi: 10.1111/bph.12226. [PMC free article] [PubMed] [CrossRef] [Google Scholar]

78. Malardé L., Groussard C., Lefeuvre-Orfila L., Vincent S., Efstathiou T., Gratas-Delamarche A. Fermented Soy Permeate Reduces Cytokine Level and Oxidative Stress in Streptozotocin-Induced Diabetic

Rats. J. Med. Food. 2015;18:67–75. doi: 10.1089/jmf.2013.0132. [PubMed] [CrossRef] [Google Scholar]

79. Tsai P.-H., Yeh C.-L., Liu J.-J., Chiu W.-C., Yeh S.-L. Effects of Dietary Glutamine on Inflammatory Mediator Gene Expressions in Rats with Streptozotocin-Induced Diabetes. Nutrition. 2012;28:288–293. doi: 10.1016/j.nut.2011.06.003. [PubMed] [CrossRef] [Google Scholar]

80. Çolak S., Geyikoğlu F., Bakır T., Türkez H., Aslan A. Evaluating the Toxic and Beneficial Effects of Lichen Extracts in Normal and Diabetic Rats. Toxicol. Ind. Health. 2016;32:1495–1504. doi: 10.1177/0748233714566873. [PubMed] [CrossRef] [Google Scholar]

81. Park J.-H., Jung J.-H., Yang J.-Y., Kim H.-S. Olive Leaf Down-Regulates the Oxidative Stress and Immune Dysregulation in Streptozotocin-Induced Diabetic Mice. Nutr. Res. 2013;33:942–951. doi: 10.1016/j.nutres.2013.07.011. [PubMed] [CrossRef] [Google Scholar]

82. Vujicic M., Nikolic I., Kontogianni V.G., Saksida T., Charisiadis P., Orescanin-Dusic Z., Blagojevic D., Stosic-Grujicic S., Tzakos A.G., Stojanovic I. Methanolic Extract of Origanum Vulgare Ameliorates Type 1 Diabetes through Antioxidant, Anti-Inflammatory and Anti-Apoptotic Activity. Br. J. Nutr. 2015;113:770–782. doi: 10.1017/S0007114514004048. [PubMed] [CrossRef] [Google Scholar]

83. Punaro G.R., Maciel F.R., Rodrigues A.M., Rogero M.M., Bogsan C.S.B., Oliveira M.N., Ihara S.S.M., Araujo S.R.R., Sanches T.R.C., Andrade L.C.,

et al. Kefir Administration Reduced Progression of Renal Injury in STZ-Diabetic Rats by Lowering Oxidative Stress. Nitric Oxide Biol. Chem. 2014;37:53–60. doi: 10.1016/j.niox.2013.12.012. [PubMed] [CrossRef] [Google Scholar]

84. Özcelik D., Nazıroglu M., Tunçdemir M., Çelik Ö., Öztürk M., Flores-Arce M.F. Zinc Supplementation Attenuates Metallothionein and Oxidative Stress Changes in Kidney of Streptozotocin-Induced Diabetic Rats. Biol. Trace Elem. Res. 2012;150:342–349. doi: 10.1007/s12011-012-9508-4. [PubMed] [CrossRef] [Google Scholar]

85. Guo Q., Wang Y., Xu D., Nossent J., Pavlos N.J., Xu J. Rheumatoid Arthritis: Pathological Mechanisms and Modern Pharmacologic Therapies. Bone Res. 2018;6:15. doi: 10.1038/s41413-018-0016-9. [PMC free article] [PubMed] [CrossRef] [Google Scholar]

86. Brennan F.M., McInnes I.B. Evidence That Cytokines Play a Role in Rheumatoid Arthritis. J. Clin. Investig. 2008;118:3537–3545. doi: 10.1172/JCI36389. [PMC free article] [PubMed] [CrossRef] [Google Scholar]

87. Scher J.U., Abramson S.B. The Microbiome and Rheumatoid Arthritis. Nat. Rev. Rheumatol. 2011;7:569. doi: 10.1038/nrrheum.2011.121. [PMC free article] [PubMed] [CrossRef] [Google Scholar]

88. Fava A., Petri M. Systemic Lupus Erythematosus: Diagnosis and Clinical Management. J. Autoimmun. 2019;96:1–13. doi: 10.1016/j.jaut.2018.11.001. [PMC free article] [PubMed] [CrossRef] [Google Scholar]

89. Parvaneh V.J., Jari M., Qhasemi S., Nasehi M.M., Rahmani K., Shiari R. Guillain–Barre Syndrome as the First Manifestation of Juvenile Systemic Lupus Erythematosus: A Case Report. Open Access Rheumatol. Res. Rev. 2019;11:97. doi: 10.2147/OARRR.S204109. [PMC free article] [PubMed] [CrossRef] [Google Scholar]

90. Beenakker E.A.C., Oparina T.I., Hartgring A., Teelken A., Arutjunyan A.V., de Keyser J. Cooling Garment Treatment in MS: Clinical Improvement and Decrease in Leukocyte NO Production. Neurology. 2001;57:892. doi: 10.1212/WNL.57.5.892. [PubMed] [CrossRef] [Google Scholar]

91. Skyrme-Jones R.A.P., O'Brien R.C., Luo M., Meredith I.T. Endothelial Vasodilator Function Is Related to Low-Density Lipoprotein Particle Size and Low-Density Lipoprotein Vitamin E Content in Type 1 Diabetes. J. Am. Coll. Cardiol. 2000;35:292–299. doi: 10.1016/S0735-1097(99)00547-1. [PubMed] [CrossRef] [Google Scholar]

92. López-Miranda J., Pérez-Jiménez F., Ros E., de Caterina R., Badimón L., Covas M.I., Escrich E., Ordovás J.M., Soriguer F., Abiá R., et al. Olive Oil and Health: Summary of the II International Conference on Olive Oil and Health Consensus Report, Jaén and Córdoba (Spain) 2008. Nutr. Metab. Cardiovasc. Dis. 2010;20:284–294. doi: 10.1016/j.numecd.2009.12.007. [PubMed] [CrossRef] [Google Scholar]

93. Franchina D.G., Dostert C., Brenner D. Reactive Oxygen Species: Involvement in T Cell Signaling and Metabolism. Trends Immunol.

2018;39:489–502. doi: 10.1016/j.it.2018.01.005. [PubMed] [CrossRef] [Google Scholar]

94. Topic A., Francuski D., Nikolic A., Milosevic K., Jovicic S., Markovic B., Djukic M., Radojkovic D. The Role of Oxidative Stress in the Clinical Manifestations of Childhood Asthma. Fetal Pediatr. Pathol. 2017;36:294–303. doi: 10.1080/15513815.2017.1315199. [PubMed] [CrossRef] [Google Scholar]

95. Venkatesha S.H., Dudics S., Astry B., Moudgil K.D. Control of Autoimmune Inflammation by Celastrol, a Natural Triterpenoid. Pathog. Dis. 2016:74. doi: 10.1093/femspd/ftw059. [PMC free article] [PubMed] [CrossRef] [Google Scholar]

96. Gianchecchi E., Fierabracci A. Insights on the Effects of Resveratrol and Some of Its Derivatives in Cancer and Autoimmunity: A Molecule with a Dual Activity. Antioxidants. 2020:9. doi: 10.3390/antiox9020091. [PMC free article] [PubMed] [CrossRef] [Google Scholar]

97. Allegra A., Musolino C., Tonacci A., Pioggia G., Gangemi S. Interactions between the MicroRNAs and Microbiota in Cancer Development: Roles and Therapeutic Opportunities. Cancers. 2020:12. doi: 10.3390/cancers12040805. [PMC free article] [PubMed] [CrossRef] [Google Scholar]

98. Casciaro M., di Salvo E., Pioggia G., Gangemi S. Microbiota and MicroRNAs in Lung Diseases: Mutual Influence and Role Insights. Eur. Rev. Med. Pharm. Sci. 2020;24:13000–13008. doi: 10.26355/eurrev_202012_24205. [PubMed] [CrossRef] [Google Scholar]

99. Constantin M.-M., Nita I.E., Olteanu R., Constantin T., Bucur S., Matei C., Raducan A. Significance and Impact of Dietary Factors on Systemic Lupus Erythematosus Pathogenesis. Exp. Med. 2019;17:1085–1090. doi: 10.3892/etm.2018.6986. [PMC free article] [PubMed] [CrossRef] [Google Scholar]

100. Petersson S., Philippou E., Rodomar C., Nikiphorou E. The Mediterranean Diet, Fish Oil Supplements and Rheumatoid Arthritis Outcomes: Evidence from Clinical Trials. Autoimmun. Rev. 2018;17:1105–1114. doi: 10.1016/j.autrev.2018.06.007. [PubMed] [CrossRef] [Google Scholar]

101. Rayess H., Wang M.B., Srivatsan E.S. Cellular Senescence and Tumor Suppressor Gene P16. Int. J. Cancer. 2012;130:1715–1725. doi: 10.1002/ijc.27316. [PMC free article] [PubMed] [CrossRef] [Google Scholar]

102. Prasad K.N. Oxidative Stress, Pro-Inflammatory Cytokines, and Antioxidants Regulate Expression Levels of MicroRNAs in Parkinson's Disease. Curr. Aging Sci. 2017;10:177–184. doi: 10.2174/1874609810666170102144233. [PubMed] [CrossRef] [Google Scholar]

103. Tavassolifar M.J., Vodjgani M., Salehi Z., Izad M. The Influence of Reactive Oxygen Species in the Immune System and Pathogenesis of Multiple Sclerosis. Autoimmune Dis. 2020;2020:5793817. doi: 10.1155/2020/5793817. [PMC free article] [PubMed] [CrossRef] [Google Scholar]

104. Tsai C.-Y., Hsieh S.-C., Lu C.-S., Wu T.-H., Liao H.-T., Wu C.-H., Li K.-J., Kuo Y.-M., Lee H.-T.,

Shen C.-Y., et al. Cross-Talk between Mitochondrial Dysfunction-Provoked Oxidative Stress and Aberrant Noncoding RNA Expression in the Pathogenesis and Pathophysiology of SLE. Int. J. Mol. Sci. 2019:20. doi: 10.3390/ijms20205183. [PMC free article] [PubMed] [CrossRef] [Google Scholar]

105. Espinós C., Galindo M.I., García-Gimeno M.A., Ibáñez-Cabellos J.S., Martínez-Rubio D., Millán J.M., Rodrigo R., Sanz P., Seco-Cervera M., Sevilla T., et al. Oxidative Stress, a Crossroad between Rare Diseases and Neurodegeneration. Antioxidants. 2020:9. doi: 10.3390/antiox9040313. [PMC free article] [PubMed] [CrossRef] [Google Scholar]

106. Birben E., Sahiner U.M., Sackesen C., Erzurum S., Kalayci O. Oxidative Stress and Antioxidant Defense. World Allergy Organ. J. 2012;5:9–19. doi: 10.1097/WOX.0b013e3182439613. [PMC free article] [PubMed] [CrossRef] [Google Scholar]

107. Baines K.J., Pavord I.D., Gibson P.G. The Role of Biomarkers in the Management of Airways Disease. Int. J. Tuberc. Lung Dis. 2014;18:1264–1268. doi: 10.5588/ijtld.14.0226. [PubMed] [CrossRef] [Google Scholar]

108. Baïz N., Chastang J., Ibanez G., Annesi-Maesano I. Prenatal Exposure to Selenium May Protect against Wheezing in Children by the Age of 3. Immun. Inflamm. Dis. 2016;5:37–44. doi: 10.1002/iid3.138. [PMC free article] [PubMed] [CrossRef] [Google Scholar]

109. Norton R.L., Hoffmann P.R. Selenium and Asthma. Mol. Asp. Med. 2012;33:98–106. doi:

10.1016/j.mam.2011.10.003. [PMC free article] [PubMed] [CrossRef] [Google Scholar]

110. Chen X., Huang Y., Feng J., Jiang X.-F., Xiao W.-F., Chen X.-X. Antioxidant and Anti-Inflammatory Effects of Schisandra and Paeonia Extracts in the Treatment of Asthma. Exp. Med. 2014;8:1479–1483. doi: 10.3892/etm.2014.1948. [PMC free article] [PubMed] [CrossRef] [Google Scholar]

111. Parthasarathy L., Khadilkar V., Chiplonkar S., Khadilkar A. Effect of Antioxidant Supplementation on Total Antioxidant Status in Indian Children with Type 1 Diabetes. J. Diet. Suppl. 2019;16:390–400. doi: 10.1080/19390211.2018.1470123. [PubMed] [CrossRef] [Google Scholar]

112. Torres-Borrego J., Moreno-Solís G., Molina-Terán A.B. Diet for the Prevention of Asthma and Allergies in Early Childhood: Much Ado about Something? Allergol. Immunopathol. 2012;40:244–252. doi: 10.1016/j.aller.2011.12.006. [PubMed] [CrossRef] [Google Scholar]

Role of collagen peptides in regulating autoimmune disease

1. Wu Y., Antony S., Meitzler J.L., Doroshow J.H. Molecular mechanisms underlying chronic inflammation-associated cancers. Cancer Lett. 2014;345:164–173. doi: 10.1016/j.canlet.2013.08.014. [PMC free article] [PubMed] [CrossRef] [Google Scholar]

2. Calder P.C., Albers R., Antoine J.M., Blum S., Bourdet-Sicard R., Ferns G.A., Folkerts G.,

Friedmann P.S., Frost G.S., Guarner F., et al. Inflammatory disease processes and interactions with nutrition. Br. J. Nutr. 2009;101:S1–S45. doi: 10.1017/S0007114509377867. [PubMed] [CrossRef] [Google Scholar]

3. Okin D., Medzhitov R. Evolution of inflammatory diseases. Curr. Biol. 2012;22:733–740. doi: 10.1016/j.cub.2012.07.029. [PMC free article] [PubMed] [CrossRef] [Google Scholar]

4. Alam Q., Alam M.Z., Mushtaq G., Damanhouri G.A., Rasool M., Kamal M.A., Haque A. Inflammatory Process in Alzheimer's and Parkinson's Diseases: Central Role of Cytokines. Curr. Pharm. Des. 2016;22:541–548. doi: 10.2174/1381612822666151125000300. [PubMed] [CrossRef] [Google Scholar]

5. Korniluk A., Koper O., Kemona H., Dymicka-Piekarska V. From inflammation to cancer. Irish J. Med. Sci. 2017;186:57–62. doi: 10.1007/s11845-016-1464-0. [PMC free article] [PubMed] [CrossRef] [Google Scholar]

6. Ouzounova M., Lee E., Piranlioglu R., El Andaloussi A., Kolhe R., Demirci M.F., Marasco D., Asm I., Chadli A., Hassan K.A., et al. Monocytic and granulocytic myeloid derived suppressor cells differentially regulate spatiotemporal tumour plasticity during metastatic cascade. Nat. Commun. 2017;8:14979. doi: 10.1038/ncomms14979. [PMC free article] [PubMed] [CrossRef] [Google Scholar]

7. Lau J.L., Dunn M.K. Therapeutic peptides: Historical perspectives, current development trends, and future directions. Bioorg. Med. Chem. 2018;26:2700–2707. doi:

10.1016/j.bmc.2017.06.052. [PubMed] [CrossRef] [Google Scholar]

8. La Manna S., Scognamiglio P.L., Di Natale C., Leone M., Mercurio F.A., Malfitano A.M., Cianfarani F., Madonna S., Caravella S., Albanesi C., et al. Characterization of linear mimetic peptides of Interleukin-22 from dissection of protein interfaces. Biochimie. 2017;138:106–115. doi: 10.1016/j.biochi.2017.05.002. [PubMed] [CrossRef] [Google Scholar]

9. Anderson P., Delgado M. Endogenous anti-inflammatory neuropeptides and pro-resolving lipid mediators: A new therapeutic approach for immune disorders. J. Cell. Mol. Med. 2008;12:1830–1847. doi: 10.1111/j.1582-4934.2008.00387.x. [PMC free article] [PubMed] [CrossRef] [Google Scholar]

10. Perretti M., Chiang N., La M., Fierro I.M., Marullo S., Getting S.J., Solito E., Serhan C.N. Endogenous lipid- and peptide-derived anti-inflammatory pathways generated with glucocorticoid and aspirin treatment activate the lipoxin A4 receptor. Nat. Med. 2002;8:1296–1302. doi: 10.1038/nm786. [PMC free article] [PubMed] [CrossRef] [Google Scholar]

11. Dietrich U., Durr R., Koch J. Peptides as drugs: From screening to application. Curr. Pharm. Biotechnol. 2013;14:501–512. doi: 10.2174/13892010113149990205. [PubMed] [CrossRef] [Google Scholar]

12. Barabasi A.L., Gulbahce N., Loscalzo J. Network medicine: A network-based approach to human disease. Nat. Rev. Genet. 2011;12:56–68. doi:

10.1038/nrg2918. [PMC free article] [PubMed] [CrossRef] [Google Scholar]

13. Flowers L.O., Johnson H.M., Mujtaba M.G., Ellis M.R., Haider S.M., Subramaniam P.S. Characterization of a peptide inhibitor of Janus kinase 2 that mimics suppressor of cytokine signaling 1 function. J. Immunol. 2004;172:7510–7518. doi: 10.4049/jimmunol.172.12.7510. [PubMed] [CrossRef] [Google Scholar]

14. Waiboci L.W., Ahmed C.M., Mujtaba M.G., Flowers L.O., Martin J.P., Haider M.I., Johnson H.M. Both the suppressor of cytokine signaling 1 (SOCS-1) kinase inhibitory region and SOCS-1 mimetic bind to JAK2 autophosphorylation site: Implications for the development of a SOCS-1 antagonist. J. Immunol. 2007;178:5058–5068. doi: 10.4049/jimmunol.178.8.5058. [PubMed] [CrossRef] [Google Scholar]

15. Doti N., Scognamiglio P.L., Madonna S., Scarponi C., Ruvo M., Perretta G., Albanesi C., Marasco D. New mimetic peptides of the kinase-inhibitory region (KIR) of SOCS1 through focused peptide libraries. Biochem. J. 2012;443:231–240. doi: 10.1042/BJ20111647. [PubMed] [CrossRef] [Google Scholar]

16. La Manna S., Lopez-Sanz L., Leone M., Brandi P., Scognamiglio P.L., Morelli G., Novellino E., Gomez-Guerrero C., Marasco D. Structure-activity studies of peptidomimetics based on kinase-inhibitory region of suppressors of cytokine signaling 1. Biopolymers. 2017 doi: 10.1002/bip.23082. [PubMed] [CrossRef] [Google Scholar]

17. La Manna S., Lee E., Ouzounova M., Di Natale C., Novellino E., Merlino A., Korkaya H., Marasco D. Mimetics of Suppressor of cytokine signalling 3: Novel potential therapeutics in triple breast cancer. Int. J. Cancer. 2018 doi: 10.1002/ijc.31594. [PubMed] [CrossRef] [Google Scholar]

18. Joshi S., Chen L., Winter M.B., Lin Y.L., Yang Y., Shapovalova M., Smith P.M., Liu C., Li F., LeBeau A.M. The Rational Design of Therapeutic Peptides for Aminopeptidase N using a Substrate-Based Approach. Sci. Rep. 2017;7:1424. doi: 10.1038/s41598-017-01542-5. [PMC free article] [PubMed] [CrossRef] [Google Scholar]

19. Eissa N., Hussein H., Kermarrec L., Grover J., Metz-Boutigue M.E., Bernstein C.N., Ghia J.E. Chromofungin Ameliorates the Progression of Colitis by Regulating Alternatively Activated Macrophages. Front. Immunol. 2017;8:1131. doi: 10.3389/fimmu.2017.01131. [PMC free article] [PubMed] [CrossRef] [Google Scholar]

20. Cobos Caceres C., Bansal P.S., Navarro S., Wilson D., Don L., Giacomin P., Loukas A., Daly N.L. An engineered cyclic peptide alleviates symptoms of inflammation in a murine model of inflammatory bowel disease. J. Biol. Chem. 2017;292:10288–10294. doi: 10.1074/jbc.M117.779215. [PMC free article] [PubMed] [CrossRef] [Google Scholar]

21. Santos A., Cabrales A., Reyes O., Gerónimo H., Rodríguez Y., Garay H., Arrieta C., Silva R., Guillén G. Identification of an interleukin-15 antagonist peptide that binds to IL-15Rα Biotecnología Aplicada. 2008;25:320–324. [Google Scholar]

22. Grundemann C., Thell K., Lengen K., Garcia-Kaufer M., Huang Y.H., Huber R., Craik D.J., Schabbauer G., Gruber C.W. Cyclotides Suppress Human T-Lymphocyte Proliferation by an Interleukin 2-Dependent Mechanism. PLoS ONE. 2013;8:e68016. doi: 10.1371/journal.pone.0068016. [PMC free article] [PubMed] [CrossRef] [Google Scholar]

23. Zellinger C., Salvamoser J.D., Seeger N., Russmann V., Potschka H. Impact of the neural cell adhesion molecule-derived peptide FGL on seizure progression and cellular alterations in the mouse kindling model. ACS Chem. Neurosci. 2014;5:185–193. doi: 10.1021/cn400153g. [PMC free article] [PubMed] [CrossRef] [Google Scholar]

24. Kurinami H., Shimamura M., Nakagami H., Shimizu H., Koriyama H., Kawano T., Wakayama K., Mochizuki H., Rakugi H., Morishita R. A Novel Therapeutic Peptide as a Partial Agonist of RANKL in Ischemic Stroke. Sci. Rep. 2016;6:38062. doi: 10.1038/srep38062. [PMC free article] [PubMed] [CrossRef] [Google Scholar]

25. Ran X., Gestwicki J.E. Inhibitors of protein-protein interactions (PPIs): An analysis of scaffold choices and buried surface area. Curr. Opin. Chem. Biol. 2018;44:75–86. doi: 10.1016/j.cbpa.2018.06.004. [PMC free article] [PubMed] [CrossRef] [Google Scholar]

26. Ciemny M., Kurcinski M., Kamel K., Kolinski A., Alam N., Schueler-Furman O., Kmiecik S. Protein-peptide docking: Opportunities and challenges. Drug Discov. Today. 2018;23:1530–1537. doi:

10.1016/j.drudis.2018.05.006. [PubMed] [CrossRef] [Google Scholar]

27. Scognamiglio P.L., Morelli G., Marasco D. Synthetic and structural routes for the rational conversion of peptides into small molecules. Methods Mol. Biol. 2015;1268:159–193. [PubMed] [Google Scholar]

28. Marasco D., Scognamiglio P.L. Identification of inhibitors of biological interactions involving intrinsically disordered proteins. Int. J. Mol. Sci. 2015;16:7394–7412. doi: 10.3390/ijms16047394. [PMC free article] [PubMed] [CrossRef] [Google Scholar]

29. Milroy L.G., Grossmann T.N., Hennig S., Brunsveld L., Ottmann C. Modulators of protein-protein interactions. Chem. Rev. 2014;114:4695–4748. doi: 10.1021/cr400698c. [PubMed] [CrossRef] [Google Scholar]

30. Mahlapuu M., Hakansson J., Ringstad L., Bjorn C. Antimicrobial Peptides: An Emerging Category of Therapeutic Agents. Front. Cell. Infect. Microbiol. 2016;6:194. doi: 10.3389/fcimb.2016.00194. [PMC free article] [PubMed] [CrossRef] [Google Scholar]

31. Roviello G.N., Vicidomini C., Costanzo V., Roviello V. Nucleic acid binding and other biomedical properties of artificial oligolysines. Int. J. Nanomed. 2016;11:5897–5904. doi: 10.2147/IJN.S121247. [PMC free article] [PubMed] [CrossRef] [Google Scholar]

32. Roviello G.N., Musumeci D., Roviello V. Cationic peptides as RNA compaction agents: A study on the polyA compaction activity of a linear alpha,

epsilon-oligo-L-lysine. Int. J. Pharm. 2015;485:244–248. doi: 10.1016/j.ijpharm.2015.03.011. [PubMed] [CrossRef] [Google Scholar]

33. O'Shea J.J., Schwartz D.M., Villarino A.V., Gadina M., McInnes I.B., Laurence A. The JAK-STAT pathway: Impact on human disease and therapeutic intervention. Annu. Rev. Med. 2015;66:311–328. doi: 10.1146/annurev-med-051113-024537. [PMC free article] [PubMed] [CrossRef] [Google Scholar]

34. Yoshimura A., Naka T., Kubo M. SOCS proteins, cytokine signalling and immune regulation. Nat. Rev. Immunol. 2007;7:454–465. doi: 10.1038/nri2093. [PubMed] [CrossRef] [Google Scholar]

35. Liang X., He M., Chen T., Liu Y., Tian Y.L., Wu Y.L., Zhao Y., Shen Y., Yuan Z.Y. Multiple roles of SOCS proteins: Differential expression of SOCS1 and SOCS3 in atherosclerosis. Int. J. Mol. Med. 2013;31:1066–1074. doi: 10.3892/ijmm.2013.1323. [PubMed] [CrossRef] [Google Scholar]

36. Kershaw N.J., Murphy J.M., Lucet I.S., Nicola N.A., Babon J.J. Regulation of Janus kinases by SOCS proteins. Biochem. Soc. Trans. 2013;41:1042–1047. doi: 10.1042/BST20130077. [PMC free article] [PubMed] [CrossRef] [Google Scholar]

37. Liau N.P.D., Laktyushin A., Lucet I.S., Murphy J.M., Yao S., Whitlock E., Callaghan K., Nicola N.A., Kershaw N.J., Babon J.J. The molecular basis of JAK-STAT inhibition by SOCS1. Nat. Commun. 2018;9:1558. doi: 10.1038/s41467-018-04013-1. [PMC free article] [PubMed] [CrossRef] [Google Scholar]

38. Shen-Orr S.S., Furman D., Kidd B.A., Hadad F., Lovelace P., Huang Y.W., Rosenberg-Hasson Y., Mackey S., Grisar F.A., Pickman Y., et al. Defective Signaling in the JAK-STAT Pathway Tracks with Chronic Inflammation and Cardiovascular Risk in Aging Humans. Cell Syst. 2016;3:374–384. doi: 10.1016/j.cels.2016.09.009. [PMC free article] [PubMed] [CrossRef] [Google Scholar]

39. Ahmed C.M., Dabelic R., Bedoya S.K., Larkin J., 3rd, Johnson H.M. A SOCS1/3 Antagonist Peptide Protects Mice Against Lethal Infection with Influenza A Virus. Front. Immunol. 2015;6:574. doi: 10.3389/fimmu.2015.00574. [PMC free article] [PubMed] [CrossRef] [Google Scholar]

40. Balabanov R., Strand K., Goswami R., McMahon E., Begolka W., Miller S.D., Popko B. Interferon-gamma-oligodendrocyte interactions in the regulation of experimental autoimmune encephalomyelitis. J. Neurosci. 2007;27:2013–2024. doi: 10.1523/JNEUROSCI.4689-06.2007. [PMC free article] [PubMed] [CrossRef] [Google Scholar]

41. Kim G., Ouzounova M., Quraishi A.A., Davis A., Tawakkol N., Clouthier S.G., Malik F., Paulson A.K., D'Angelo R.C., Korkaya S., et al. SOCS3-mediated regulation of inflammatory cytokines in PTEN and p53 inactivated triple negative breast cancer model. Oncogene. 2015;34:671–680. doi: 10.1038/onc.2014.4. [PMC free article] [PubMed] [CrossRef] [Google Scholar]

42. Linossi E.M., Babon J.J., Hilton D.J., Nicholson S.E. Suppression of cytokine signaling: The SOCS perspective. Cytokine Growth Factor Rev. 2013;24:241–248. doi:

10.1016/j.cytogfr.2013.03.005. [PMC free article] [PubMed] [CrossRef] [Google Scholar]

43. Trengove M.C., Ward A.C. SOCS proteins in development and disease. Am. J. Clin. Exp. Immunol. 2013;2:1–29. [PMC free article] [PubMed] [Google Scholar]

44. Flowers L.O., Subramaniam P.S., Johnson H.M. A SOCS-1 peptide mimetic inhibits both constitutive and IL-6 induced activation of STAT3 in prostate cancer cells. Oncogene. 2005;24:2114–2120. doi: 10.1038/sj.onc.1208437. [PubMed] [CrossRef] [Google Scholar]

45. Ahmed C.M., Dabelic R., Waiboci L.W., Jager L.D., Heron L.L., Johnson H.M. SOCS-1 mimetics protect mice against lethal poxvirus infection: Identification of a novel endogenous antiviral system. J. Virol. 2009;83:1402–1415. doi: 10.1128/JVI.01138-08. [PMC free article] [PubMed] [CrossRef] [Google Scholar]

46. Mujtaba M.G., Flowers L.O., Patel C.B., Patel R.A., Haider M.I., Johnson H.M. Treatment of mice with the suppressor of cytokine signaling-1 mimetic peptide, tyrosine kinase inhibitor peptide, prevents development of the acute form of experimental allergic encephalomyelitis and induces stable remission in the chronic relapsing/remitting form. J. Immunol. 2005;175:5077–5086. [PubMed] [Google Scholar]

47. Madonna S., Scarponi C., Morelli M., Sestito R., Scognamiglio P.L., Marasco D., Albanesi C. SOCS3 inhibits the pathological effects of IL-22 in non-melanoma skin tumor-derived keratinocytes. Oncotarget. 2017;8:24652–24667. doi:

10.18632/oncotarget.15629. [PMC free article] [PubMed] [CrossRef] [Google Scholar]

48. Madonna S., Scarponi C., Doti N., Carbone T., Cavani A., Scognamiglio P.L., Marasco D., Albanesi C. Therapeutical potential of a peptide mimicking the SOCS1 kinase inhibitory region in skin immune responses. Eur. J. Immunol. 2013;43:1883–1895. doi: 10.1002/eji.201343370. [PubMed] [CrossRef] [Google Scholar]

49. Williams G., Eickholt B.J., Maison P., Prinjha R., Walsh F.S., Doherty P. A complementary peptide approach applied to the design of novel semaphorin/neuropilin antagonists. J. Neurochem. 2005;92:1180–1190. doi: 10.1111/j.1471-4159.2004.02950.x. [PubMed] [CrossRef] [Google Scholar]

50. Decaffmeyer M., Lins L., Charloteaux B., VanEyck M.H., Thomas A., Brasseur R. Rational design of complementary peptides to the betaAmyloid 29-42 fusion peptide: An application of PepDesign. Biochim. Biophys. Acta. 2006;1758:320–327. doi: 10.1016/j.bbamem.2005.10.001. [PubMed] [CrossRef] [Google Scholar]

51. Ahmed C.M., Larkin J., 3rd, Johnson H.M. SOCS1 Mimetics and Antagonists: A Complementary Approach to Positive and Negative Regulation of Immune Function. Front. Immunol. 2015;6:183. doi: 10.3389/fimmu.2015.00183. [PMC free article] [PubMed] [CrossRef] [Google Scholar]

52. Recio C., Oguiza A., Lazaro I., Mallavia B., Egido J., Gomez-Guerrero C. Suppressor of cytokine signaling 1-derived peptide inhibits Janus kinase/signal transducers and activators of

transcription pathway and improves inflammation and atherosclerosis in diabetic mice. Arterioscler. Thromb. Vasc. Biol. 2014;34:1953–1960. doi: 10.1161/ATVBAHA.114.304144. [PubMed] [CrossRef] [Google Scholar]

53. Recio C., Lazaro I., Oguiza A., Lopez-Sanz L., Bernal S., Blanco J., Egido J., Gomez-Guerrero C. Suppressor of Cytokine Signaling-1 Peptidomimetic Limits Progression of Diabetic Nephropathy. J. Am. Soc. Nephrol. 2017;28:575–585. doi: 10.1681/ASN.2016020237. [PMC free article] [PubMed] [CrossRef] [Google Scholar]

54. Marasco D., Perretta G., Sabatella M., Ruvo M. Past and Future Perspectives of Synthetic Peptide Libraries. Curr. Protein Pept. Sci. 2008;9:447–467. doi: 10.2174/138920308785915209. [PubMed] [CrossRef] [Google Scholar]

55. Humet M., Carbonell T., Masip I., Sanchez-Baeza F., Mora P., Canton E., Gobernado M., Abad C., Perez-Paya E., Messeguer A. A positional scanning combinatorial library of peptoids as a source of biological active molecules: Identification of antimicrobials. J. Comb. Chem. 2003;5:597–605. doi: 10.1021/cc020075u. [PubMed] [CrossRef] [Google Scholar]

56. Madonna S., Scarponi C., Sestito R., Doti N., Carbone T., Nasorri F., Marasco D., Cavani A., Albanesi C. Mimetic peptides of suppressor of cytokine signaling (SOCS)1 impair inflammatory responses of epidermal keratinocytes in vitro and in a mouse skin model of allergic contact dermatitis. J. Investig. Dermatol. 2011;131:S11. [Google Scholar]

57. Korkaya H., Kim G.I., Davis A., Malik F., Henry N.L., Ithimakin S., Quraishi A.A., Tawakkol N., D'Angelo R., Paulson A.K., et al. Activation of an IL6 inflammatory loop mediates trastuzumab resistance in HER2+ breast cancer by expanding the cancer stem cell population. Mol. Cell. 2012;47:570–584. doi: 10.1016/j.molcel.2012.06.014. [PMC free article] [PubMed] [CrossRef] [Google Scholar]

58. Inagaki-Ohara K., Kondo T., Ito M., Yoshimura A. SOCS, inflammation, and cancer. Jakstat. 2013;2:e24053. doi: 10.4161/jkst.24053. [PMC free article] [PubMed] [CrossRef] [Google Scholar]

59. Kershaw N.J., Murphy J.M., Liau N.P., Varghese L.N., Laktyushin A., Whitlock E.L., Lucet I.S., Nicola N.A., Babon J.J. SOCS3 binds specific receptor-JAK complexes to control cytokine signaling by direct kinase inhibition. Nat. Struct. Mol. Biol. 2013;20:469–476. doi: 10.1038/nsmb.2519. [PMC free article] [PubMed] [CrossRef] [Google Scholar]

60. Mucha A., Drag M., Dalton J.P., Kafarski P. Metallo-aminopeptidase inhibitors. Biochimie. 2010;92:1509–1529. doi: 10.1016/j.biochi.2010.04.026. [PMC free article] [PubMed] [CrossRef] [Google Scholar]

61. Drinkwater N., Lee J., Yang W., Malcolm T.R., McGowan S. M1 aminopeptidases as drug targets: Broad applications or therapeutic niche? FEBS J. 2017;284:1473–1488. doi: 10.1111/febs.14009. [PMC free article] [PubMed] [CrossRef] [Google Scholar]

62. Ito K., Nakajima Y., Onohara Y., Takeo M., Nakashima K., Matsubara F., Ito T., Yoshimoto T. Crystal structure of aminopeptidase N

(proteobacteria alanyl aminopeptidase) from Escherichia coli and conformational change of methionine 260 involved in substrate recognition. J. Biol. Chem. 2006;281:33664–33676. doi: 10.1074/jbc.M605203200. [PubMed] [CrossRef] [Google Scholar]

63. Wickstrom M., Larsson R., Nygren P., Gullbo J. Aminopeptidase N (CD13) as a target for cancer chemotherapy. Cancer Sci. 2011;102:501–508. doi: 10.1111/j.1349-7006.2010.01826.x. [PMC free article] [PubMed] [CrossRef] [Google Scholar]

64. Keyal U., Liu Y., Bhatta A.K. Dermatologic manifestations of inflammatory bowel disease: A review. Discov. Med. 2018;25:225–233. [PubMed] [Google Scholar]

65. Bain C.C., Mowat A.M. Macrophages in intestinal homeostasis and inflammation. Immunol. Rev. 2014;260:102–117. doi: 10.1111/imr.12192. [PMC free article] [PubMed] [CrossRef] [Google Scholar]

66. Karrasch T., Jobin C. NF-kappaB and the intestine: Friend or foe? Inflamm. Bowel. Dis. 2008;14:114–124. doi: 10.1002/ibd.20243. [PubMed] [CrossRef] [Google Scholar]

67. Loh Y.P., Cheng Y., Mahata S.K., Corti A., Tota B. Chromogranin A and derived peptides in health and disease. J. Mol. Neurosci. 2012;48:347–356. doi: 10.1007/s12031-012-9728-2. [PMC free article] [PubMed] [CrossRef] [Google Scholar]

68. D'Amico M.A., Ghinassi B., Izzicupo P., Manzoli L., Di Baldassarre A. Biological function and clinical relevance of chromogranin A and derived peptides. Endocr. Connect. 2014;3:R45–R54. doi:

10.1530/EC-14-0027. [PMC free article] [PubMed] [CrossRef] [Google Scholar]

69. Eissa N., Hussein H., Kermarrec L., Elgazzar O., Metz-Boutigue M.H., Bernstein C.N., Ghia J.E. Chromofungin (CHR: CHGA47-66) is downregulated in persons with active ulcerative colitis and suppresses pro-inflammatory macrophage function through the inhibition of NF-kappaB signaling. Biochem. Pharmacol. 2017;145:102–113. doi: 10.1016/j.bcp.2017.08.013. [PubMed] [CrossRef] [Google Scholar]

70. Novak M.L., Koh T.J. Macrophage phenotypes during tissue repair. J. Leukoc. Biol. 2013;93:875–881. doi: 10.1189/jlb.1012512. [PMC free article] [PubMed] [CrossRef] [Google Scholar]

71. Liu T., Zhang L., Joo D., Sun S.C. NF-kappaB signaling in inflammation. Signal. Transduct. Target Ther. 2017;2:17023. doi: 10.1038/sigtrans.2017.23. [PMC free article] [PubMed] [CrossRef] [Google Scholar]

72. Grzanka A., Misiolek M., Golusinski W., Jarzab J. Molecular mechanisms of glucocorticoids action: Implications for treatment of rhinosinusitis and nasal polyposis. Eur. Arch. Oto-Rhino-L. 2011;268:247–253. doi: 10.1007/s00405-010-1330-z. [PMC free article] [PubMed] [CrossRef] [Google Scholar]

73. Ouyang N., Zhu C., Zhou D., Nie T., Go M.F., Richards R.J., Rigas B. MC-12, an annexin A1-based peptide, is effective in the treatment of experimental colitis. PLoS ONE. 2012;7:e41585. doi: 10.1371/journal.pone.0041585. [PMC free article] [PubMed] [CrossRef] [Google Scholar]

74. Bruschi M., Petretto A., Vaglio A., Santucci L., Candiano G., Ghiggeri G.M. Annexin A1 and Autoimmunity: From Basic Science to Clinical Applications. Int. J. Mol. Sci. 2018;19:1348. doi: 10.3390/ijms19051348. [PMC free article] [PubMed] [CrossRef] [Google Scholar]

75. Scannell M., Flanagan M.B., deStefani A., Wynne K.J., Cagney G., Godson C., Maderna P. Annexin-1 and peptide derivatives are released by apoptotic cells and stimulate phagocytosis of apoptotic neutrophils by macrophages. J. Immunol. 2007;178:4595–4605. doi: 10.4049/jimmunol.178.7.4595. [PubMed] [CrossRef] [Google Scholar]

76. Zhang Z., Huang L., Zhao W., Rigas B. Annexin 1 induced by anti-inflammatory drugs binds to NF-kappaB and inhibits its activation: Anticancer effects in vitro and in vivo. Cancer Res. 2010;70:2379–2388. doi: 10.1158/0008-5472.CAN-09-4204. [PMC free article] [PubMed] [CrossRef] [Google Scholar]

77. Villadsen L.S., Schuurman J., Beurskens F., Dam T.N., Dagnaes-Hansen F., Skov L., Rygaard J., Voorhorst-Ogink M.M., Gerritsen A.F., van Dijk M.A., et al. Resolution of psoriasis upon blockade of IL-15 biological activity in a xenograft mouse model. J. Clin. Investig. 2003;112:1571–1580. doi: 10.1172/JCI200318986. [PMC free article] [PubMed] [CrossRef] [Google Scholar]

78. Giri J.G., Kumaki S., Ahdieh M., Friend D.J., Loomis A., Shanebeck K., DuBose R., Cosman D., Park L.S., Anderson D.M. Identification and cloning of a novel IL-15 binding protein that is structurally related to the alpha chain of the IL-2 receptor. EMBO

J. 1995;14:3654–3663. doi: 10.1002/j.1460-2075.1995.tb00035.x. [PMC free article] [PubMed] [CrossRef] [Google Scholar]

79. Abadie V., Jabri B. IL-15: A central regulator of celiac disease immunopathology. Immunol. Rev. 2014;260:221–234. doi: 10.1111/imr.12191. [PMC free article] [PubMed] [CrossRef] [Google Scholar]

80. Savio A.S., Acosta O.R., Perez H.G., Alvarez Y.R., Chico A., Ojeda M.O., Aguero C.A., Estevez M., Nieto G.G. Enhancement of the inhibitory effect of an IL-15 antagonist peptide by alanine scanning. J. Pept. Sci. 2012;18:25–29. doi: 10.1002/psc.1411. [PubMed] [CrossRef] [Google Scholar]

81. Rodriguez-Alvarez Y., Cabrales-Rico A., Perera-Pintado A., Prats-Capote A., Garay-Perez H.E., Reyes-Acosta O., Perez-Garcia E., Chico-Capote A., Santos-Savio A. In vitro and in vivo characterization of an interleukin-15 antagonist peptide by metabolic stability, Tc-99m-labeling, and biological activity assays. J. Pept. Sci. 2018;24:e3078. doi: 10.1002/psc.3078. [PubMed] [CrossRef] [Google Scholar]

82. Yang X.K., Xu W.D., Leng R.X., Liang Y., Liu Y.Y., Fang X.Y., Feng C.C., Li R., Cen H., Pan H.F., et al. Therapeutic potential of IL-15 in rheumatoid arthritis. Hum. Immunol. 2015;76:812–818. doi: 10.1016/j.humimm.2015.09.041. [PubMed] [CrossRef] [Google Scholar]

83. Simonsen S.M., Sando L., Rosengren K.J., Wang C.K., Colgrave M.L., Daly N.L., Craik D.J. Alanine scanning mutagenesis of the prototypic cyclotide reveals a cluster of residues essential for bioactivity. J. Biol. Chem. 2008;283:9805–9813. doi:

10.1074/jbc.M709303200. [PubMed] [CrossRef] [Google Scholar]

84. Huang Y.H., Colgrave M.L., Clark R.J., Kotze A.C., Craik D.J. Lysine-scanning mutagenesis reveals an amendable face of the cyclotide kalata B1 for the optimization of nematocidal activity. J. Biol. Chem. 2010;285:10797–10805. doi: 10.1074/jbc.M109.089854. [PMC free article] [PubMed] [CrossRef] [Google Scholar]

85. Thell K., Hellinger R., Sahin E., Michenthaler P., Gold-Binder M., Haider T., Kuttke M., Liutkeviciute Z., Goransson U., Grundemann C., et al. Oral activity of a nature-derived cyclic peptide for the treatment of multiple sclerosis. Proc. Natl. Acad. Sci. USA. 2016;113:3960–3965. doi: 10.1073/pnas.1519960113. [PMC free article] [PubMed] [CrossRef] [Google Scholar]

86. Gadani S.P., Cronk J.C., Norris G.T., Kipnis J. IL-4 in the Brain: A Cytokine To Remember. J. Immunol. 2012;189:4213–4219. doi: 10.4049/jimmunol.1202246. [PMC free article] [PubMed] [CrossRef] [Google Scholar]

87. Russo A., Aiello C., Grieco P., Marasco D. Targeting 'Undruggable' Proteins: Design of Synthetic Cyclopeptides. Curr. Med. Chem. 2016;23:748–762. doi: 10.2174/0929867323666160112122540. [PubMed] [CrossRef] [Google Scholar]

88. Kiselyov V.V., Skladchikova G., Hinsby A.M., Jensen P.H., Kulahin N., Soroka V., Pedersen N., Tsetlin V., Poulsen F.M., Berezin V., et al. Structural basis for a direct interaction between FGFR1 and NCAM and evidence for a regulatory role of ATP.

Structure. 2003;11:691–701. doi: 10.1016/S0969-2126(03)00096-0. [PubMed] [CrossRef] [Google Scholar]

89. Secher T., Novitskaia V., Berezin V., Bock E., Glenthoj B., Klementiev B. A neural cell adhesion molecule-derived fibroblast growth factor receptor agonist, the FGL-peptide, promotes early postnatal sensorimotor development and enhances social memory retention. Neuroscience. 2006;141:1289–1299. doi: 10.1016/j.neuroscience.2006.04.059. [PubMed] [CrossRef] [Google Scholar]

90. Aonurm-Helm A., Berezin V., Bock E., Zharkovsky A. NCAM-mimetic, FGL peptide, restores disrupted fibroblast growth factor receptor (FGFR) phosphorylation and FGFR mediated signaling in neural cell adhesion molecule (NCAM)-deficient mice. Brain Res. 2010;1309:1–8. doi: 10.1016/j.brainres.2009.11.003. [PubMed] [CrossRef] [Google Scholar]

91. Downer E.J., Cowley T.R., Lyons A., Mills K.H., Berezin V., Bock E., Lynch M.A. A novel anti-inflammatory role of NCAM-derived mimetic peptide, FGL. Neurobiol. Aging. 2010;31:118–128. doi: 10.1016/j.neurobiolaging.2008.03.017. [PubMed] [CrossRef] [Google Scholar]

92. Asua D., Bougamra G., Calleja-Felipe M., Morales M., Knafo S. Peptides Acting as Cognitive Enhancers. Neuroscience. 2018;370:81–87. doi: 10.1016/j.neuroscience.2017.10.002. [PubMed] [CrossRef] [Google Scholar]

93. Lakhan S.E., Kirchgessner A., Hofer M. Inflammatory mechanisms in ischemic stroke: Therapeutic approaches. J. Transl. Med. 2009;7:97.

doi: 10.1186/1479-5876-7-97. [PMC free article] [PubMed] [CrossRef] [Google Scholar]

94. Doti N., Reuther C., Scognamiglio P.L., Dolga A.M., Plesnila N., Ruvo M., Culmsee C. Inhibition of the AIF/CypA complex protects against intrinsic death pathways induced by oxidative stress. Cell Death Dis. 2014;5:e993. doi: 10.1038/cddis.2013.518. [PMC free article] [PubMed] [CrossRef] [Google Scholar]

95. Shimamura M., Nakagami H., Osako M.K., Kurinami H., Koriyama H., Zhengda P., Tomioka H., Tenma A., Wakayama K., Morishita R. OPG/RANKL/RANK axis is a critical inflammatory signaling system in ischemic brain in mice. Proc. Natl. Acad. Sci. USA. 2014;111:8191–8196. doi: 10.1073/pnas.1400544111. [PMC free article] [PubMed] [CrossRef] [Google Scholar]

General Overviews on Stress and Autoimmune Disease

1. Cohen, S., Janicki-Deverts, D., & Miller, G. E. (2007). Psychological stress and disease. JAMA, 298(14), 1685-1687.

2. Dhabhar, F. S. (2014). Effects of stress on immune function: The good, the bad, and the beautiful. Immunologic Research, 58, 193-210.

3. Padgett, D. A., & Glaser, R. (2003). How stress influences the immune response. Trends in Immunology, 24(8), 444-448.

4. Bierhaus, A., Wolf, J., Andrassy, M., et al. (2003). A mechanism converting psychosocial stress into mononuclear cell activation. PNAS, 100(4), 1920-1925.

Cortisol and HPA Axis in Autoimmunity

5. Tsigos, C., & Chrousos, G. P. (2002). Hypothalamic–pituitary–adrenal axis, neuroendocrine factors, and stress. Journal of Psychosomatic Research, 53(4), 865-871.

6. Selye, H. (1976). The Stress of Life. McGraw-Hill.
A foundational text on the stress response and its relationship to health, including immune-mediated diseases.

Specific Autoimmune Diseases and Stress

7. Lupus:
Stojanovich, L., & Marisavljevich, D. (2008). Stress as a trigger of autoimmune disease. Autoimmunity Reviews, 7(3), 209-213.

8. Multiple Sclerosis:
Mohr, D. C., Hart, S. L., Julian, L., Cox, D., & Pelletier, D. (2004). Association between stressful life events and exacerbation in multiple sclerosis: A meta-analysis. BMJ, 328(7442), 731.

9. Zhang, T. Y., & Meaney, M. J. (2010). Epigenetics and the environmental regulation of the genome and its function. Annual Review of Psychology, 61, 439-466.

10. Cohen, I. R. (2000). Tending Adam's Garden: Evolving the Cognitive Immune Self. Academic Press.

11. Segerstrom, S. C., & Miller, G. E. (2004). Psychological stress and the human immune system: A meta-analytic study of 30 years of inquiry. Psychological Bulletin, 130(4), 601-630.

12. Jiang, L., et al. (2018). The role of stress in the development of autoimmune diseases: A review. Autoimmunity Reviews, 17(7), 665-676.

13. Sapolsky, R. M., Romero, L. M., & Munck, A. U. (2000). How do glucocorticoids influence stress

responses? Integrating permissive, suppressive, stimulatory, and preparative actions. Endocrine Reviews, 21(1), 55-89.

14. Godbout, J. P., & Glaser, R. (2006). Stress-induced immune dysregulation: Implications for wound healing, infectious disease and cancer. Journal of Neuroimmune Pharmacology, 1(4), 421-427.

15. Chrousos, G. P. (2009). Stress and disorders of the stress system. Nature Reviews Endocrinology, 5(7), 374-381.

16. Silverman, M. N., Pearce, B. D., Biron, C. A., & Miller, A. H. (2005). Immune modulation of the hypothalamic-pituitary-adrenal (HPA) axis during viral infection. Viral Immunology, 18(1), 41-78.

17. Ader, R., Cohen, N., & Felten, D. (1995). Psychoneuroimmunology: Interactions between the nervous system and the immune system. The Lancet, 345(8942), 99-103.

18. Ader, R. (Ed.). (2007). Psychoneuroimmunology (4th ed.). Academic Press.

19. Rabin, B. S. (1999). Stress, Immune Function, and Health: The Connection. Wiley-Liss.

20. Goldman, L. Cecil Medicine, Saunders, 2007.

21. Firestein, G. Kelley's Textbook of Rheumatology, W.B. Saunders Company, 2008.

22. Acta Myologica: 'Giant cell myositis and myocarditis revisited.'

23. Boston Children's Hospital: 'Autoimmune Diseases.'

24. Center for Autoimmune Neurology: 'Anti-NMDAR Encephalitis.'

25. Cleveland Clinic: 'Autoimmune Diseases.'

26. John Hopkins Medicine: 'Autoimmune Disease: Why Is My Immune System Attacking Itself?,' 'What Are Common Symptoms of Autoimmune Disease?'

27. Mayo Clinic: 'Mixed connective tissue disease.'

28. MedlinePlus: 'Autoimmune disorders,' '5 common autoimmune diseases,' 'Autoimmune diseases.'

29. Mount Sinai: 'Autoimmune disorders.'

30. National Institutes of Health: 'Understanding Autoimmune Diseases.'

31. National Stem Cell Foundation: 'Autoimmune Disease.'

32. Office on Women's Health: 'Autoimmune Diseases.'

33. Penn Medicine: 'Amanda's Story About Anti-NMDA Receptor Encephalitis.'

34. National Institute of Environmental Health Sciences: 'Autoimmune Diseases.'

35. Global Autoimmune Institute: 'Autoimmune Disease Basics.'

36. National Eczema Association: 'Is Eczema an Autoimmune Disease? Spoiler Alert: Nope.'

TRIGGERS

1. Stress as a trigger of autoimmune disease.
Stojanovich L, et al. Autoimmun Rev. 2008. PMID: 18190880 Review.

3. Lupus and other autoimmune diseases: Epidemiology in the population of African ancestry and diagnostic and management challenges in Africa.
Essouma M, et al. J Allergy Clin Immunol Glob. 2024. PMID: 39282618 Free PMC article. Review.

4. Autoimmune Diseases Following Environmental Disasters: A Narrative Review of the Literature.
Mpakosi A, et al. Healthcare (Basel). 2024. PMID: 39273791 Free PMC article. Review.

5. Pregnancy complications and new-onset maternal autoimmune disease.
Scime NV, et al. Int J Epidemiol. 2024. PMID: 39191479 Free PMC article.

6. Nanomedicines Targeting Ferroptosis to Treat Stress-Related Diseases.
Kang H, et al. Int J Nanomedicine. 2024. PMID: 39157732 Free PMC article. Review.

7. Higher Rates of Certain Autoimmune Diseases in Transgender and Gender Diverse Youth.
Logel SN, et al. Transgend Health. 2024. PMID: 39109261

8.Efficacy of substances containing 3 types of active ingredients-saponins, flavones, and alkaloids in regulation of cytokines in autoimmune diseases a systematic review and Meta-analysis based on animal studies.
Ruifang Z, et al. J Tradit Chin Med. 2024. PMID: 38767625 Free PMC article.

9.Antiphospholipid syndrome presenting as extensive skin ulcers on unilateral lower extremity: a case report.
Yang Y, et al. Front Surg. 2024. PMID: 38660586 Free PMC article.

10.An intersectionality framework for identifying relevant covariates in health equity research.
Simkus A, et al. Front Public Health. 2024. PMID: 38560446 Free PMC article. Review.

1.Stress as a trigger of autoimmune disease.
Stojanovich L, et al. Autoimmun Rev. 2008. PMID: 18190880 Review.

2.Semen adaptation to microbes in an insect.
Otti O, et al. Evol Lett. 2024. PMID: 39328283 Free PMC article.

3.Lupus and other autoimmune diseases: Epidemiology in the population of African ancestry and diagnostic and management challenges in Africa.
Essouma M, et al. J Allergy Clin Immunol Glob. 2024. PMID: 39282618 Free PMC article. Review.

4.Autoimmune Diseases Following Environmental Disasters: A Narrative Review of the Literature.
Mpakosi A, et al. Healthcare (Basel). 2024. PMID: 39273791 Free PMC article. Review.

5.Pregnancy complications and new-onset maternal autoimmune disease.
Scime NV, et al. Int J Epidemiol. 2024. PMID: 39191479 Free PMC article.

6.Nanomedicines Targeting Ferroptosis to Treat Stress-Related Diseases.
Kang H, et al. Int J Nanomedicine. 2024. PMID: 39157732 Free PMC article. Review.

7.Higher Rates of Certain Autoimmune Diseases in Transgender and Gender Diverse Youth.
Logel SN, et al. Transgend Health. 2024. PMID: 39109261

8.Efficacy of substances containing 3 types of active ingredients-saponins, flavones, and alkaloids in regulation of cytokines in autoimmune diseases a systematic review and Meta-analysis based on animal studies.
Ruifang Z, et al. J Tradit Chin Med. 2024. PMID: 38767625 Free PMC article.

9.Antiphospholipid syndrome presenting as extensive skin ulcers on unilateral lower extremity: a case report.
Yang Y, et al. Front Surg. 2024. PMID: 38660586 Free PMC article.

10.An intersectionality framework for identifying relevant covariates in health equity research.
Simkus A, et al. Front Public Health. 2024. PMID: 38560446 Free PMC article. Review.

11.Effect of radiotherapy on head and neck cancer tissues in patients receiving radiotherapy: a bioinformatics analysis-based study.
Guan Z, et al. Sci Rep. 2024. PMID: 38491080 Free PMC article.

12.Chronic social stress in early life can predispose mice to antisocial maltreating behavior.
Jeon D, et al. Encephalitis. 2024. PMID: 38444108 Free PMC article.

13.Immunologic derangement caused by intestinal dysbiosis and stress is the intrinsic basis of reactive arthritis.
He T, et al. Z Rheumatol. 2024. PMID: 38403666 Review. English.

14.Restoring immune tolerance in pemphigus vulgaris.
Ahmed AR, et al. Proc Natl Acad Sci U S A. 2024. PMID: 38261616 Free PMC article.

15.Evaluation of the benefits of neutral bicarbonate ionized water baths in an open-label, randomized, crossover trial.
Ushikoshi-Nakayama R, et al. Sci Rep. 2024. PMID: 38218992 Free PMC article. Clinical Trial.

16. Pemphigus: trigger and predisposing factors.
Moro F, et al. Front Med (Lausanne). 2023. PMID: 38213911 Free PMC article. Review.

17. Effect of electroacupuncture at Neiguan (PC6) at different time points on myocardial ischemia reperfusion arrhythmia in rats.
Qianhui S, et al. J Tradit Chin Med. 2024. PMID: 38213246 Free PMC article.

18. Applications of cold atmospheric plasma in immune-mediated inflammatory diseases via redox homeostasis: evidence and prospects.
Ma Y, et al. Heliyon. 2023. PMID: 38107323 Free PMC article.

19. The Role of Small Airway Disease in Pulmonary Fibrotic Diseases.
Barkas GI, et al. J Pers Med. 2023. PMID: 38003915 Free PMC article. Review.

20. Stress, psychiatric disease, and obesity: An Obesity Medicine Association (OMA) Clinical Practice Statement (CPS) 2022.
Christensen SM, et al. Obes Pillars. 2022. PMID: 37990662 Free PMC article.

21. Theoharides, T. C. (2020). Stress, Inflammation, and Autoimmunity: The 3 Modern Erinyes. Clinical Therapeutics, 42(5), 742-744. https://doi.org/10.1016/j.clinthera.2020.04.002